MindBody Medicine

ROUTLEDGE PSYCHOSOCIAL STRESS SERIES

Charles R. Figley, Ph.D., Series Editor

1. *Stress Disorders among Vietnam Veterans*, Edited by Charles R. Figley, Ph.D.
2. *Stress and the Family Vol. 1: Coping with Normative Transitions*, Edited by Hamilton I. McCubbin, Ph.D., and Charles R. Figley, Ph.D.
3. *Stress and the Family Vol. 2: Coping with Catastrophe*, Edited by Charles R. Figley, Ph.D., and Hamilton I. McCubbin, Ph.D.
4. *Trauma and Its Wake: The Study and Treatment of Post-Traumatic Stress Disorder*, Edited by Charles R. Figley, Ph.D.
5. *Post-Traumatic Stress Disorder and the War Veteran Patient*, Edited by William E. Kelly, M.D.
6. *The Crime Victim's Book, Second Edition*, by Morton Bard, Ph.D., and Dawn Sangrey.
7. *Stress and Coping in Time of War: Generalizations from the Israeli Experience*, Edited by Norman A. Milgram, Ph.D.
8. *Trauma and Its Wake Vol. 2: Traumatic Stress Theory, Research, and Intervention*, Edited by Charles R. Figley, Ph.D.
9. *Stress and Addiction*, Edited by Edward Gottheil, M.D., Ph.D., Keith A. Druley, Ph.D., Steven Pashko, Ph.D., and Stephen P. Weinsteinn, Ph.D.
10. *Vietnam: A Casebook*, by Jacob D. Lindy, M.D., in collaboration with Bonnie L. Green, Ph.D., Mary C. Grace, M.Ed., M.S., John A. MacLeod, M.D., and Louis Spitz, M.D.
11. *Post-Traumatic Therapy and Victims of Violence*, Edited by Frank M. Ochberg, M.D.
12. *Mental Health Response to Mass Emergencies: Theory and Practice*, Edited by Mary Lystad, Ph.D.
13. *Treating Stress in Families*, Edited by Charles R. Figley, Ph.D.
14. *Trauma, Transformation, and Healing: An Integrative Approach to Theory, Research, and Post-Traumatic Therapy*, by John P. Wilson, Ph.D.
15. *Systemic Treatment of Incest: A Therapeutic Handbook*, by Terry Trepper, Ph.D., and Mary Jo Barrett, M.S.W.
16. *The Crisis of Competence: Transitional Stress and the Displaced Worker*, Edited by Carl A. Maida, Ph.D., Norma S. Gordon, M.A., and Norman L. Farberow, Ph.D.
17. *Stress Management: An Integrated Approach to Therapy*, by Dorothy H. G. Cotton, Ph.D.
18. *Trauma and the Vietnam War Generation: Report of the Findings from the National Vietnam Veterans Readjustment Study*, by Richard A. Kulka, Ph.D., William E. Schlenger, Ph.D., John A. Fairbank, Ph.D., Richard L. Hough, Ph.D., Kathleen Jordan, Ph.D., Charles R. Marmar, M.D., Daniel S. Weiss, Ph.D., and David A. Grady, Psy.D.
19. *Strangers at Home: Vietnam Veterans Since the War*, Edited by Charles R. Figley, Ph.D., and Seymour Leventman, Ph.D.
20. *The National Vietnam Veterans Readjustment Study: Tables of Findings and Technical Appendices*, by Richard A. Kulka, Ph.D., Kathleen Jordan, Ph.D., Charles R. Marmar, M.D., and Daniel S. Weiss, Ph.D.
21. *Psychological Trauma and the Adult Survivor: Theory, Therapy, and Transformation*, by I. Lisa McCann, Ph.D., and Laurie Anne Pearlman, Ph.D.
22. *Coping with Infant or Fetal Loss: The Couple's Healing Process*, by Kathleen R. Gilbert, Ph.D., and Laura S. Smart, Ph.D.
23. *Compassion Fatigue: Coping with Secondary Traumatic Stress Disorder in Those Who Treat the Traumatized*, Edited by Charles R. Figley, Ph.D.
24. *Treating Compassion Fatigue*, Edited by Charles R. Figley, Ph.D.
25. *Handbook of Stress, Trauma and the Family*, Edited by Don R. Catherall, Ph.D.
26. *The Pain of Helping: Psychological Injury of Helping Professionals*, by Patrick J. Morrissette, Ph.D., RMFT, NCC, CCC.
27. *Disaster Mental Health Services: A Primer for Practitioners*, by Diane Myers, R.N., M.S.N., and David Wee, M.S.S.W.
28. *Empathy in the Treatment of Trauma and PTSD*, by John P. Wilson, Ph.D. and Rhiannon B. Thomas, Ph.D.
29. *Family Stressors: Interventions for Stress and Trauma*, Edited by Don. R. Catherall, Ph. D.
30. *Handbook of Women, Stress and Trauma*, Edited by Kathleen Kendall-Tackett, Ph.D.
31. *Mapping Trauma and Its Wake*, Edited by Charles R. Figley, Ph.D.
32. *The Posttraumatic Self: Restoring Meaning and Wholeness to Personality*, Edited by John P. Wilson, Ph.D.
33. *Violent Death: Resilience and Intervention Beyond the Crisis*, Edited by Edward K. Rynearson, M.D.
34. *Combat Stress Injury: Theory, Research, and Management*, Edited by Charles R. Figly, Ph.D. and William P. Nash, M.D.

EDITORIAL BOARD

MindBody Medicine

Foundations and Practical Applications

Leo W. Rotan
Veronika Ospina-Kammerer

Routledge
Taylor & Francis Group
NEW YORK AND LONDON

Routledge
Taylor & Francis Group
711 Third Avenue,
New York, NY 10017

Routledge
Taylor & Francis Group
2 Park Square, Milton Park,
Abingdon, Oxfordshire OX14 4RN

First issued in paperback 2015

Routledge is an imprint of the Taylor and Francis Group, an informa business

ISBN 13: 978-1-138-99588-8 (pbk)
ISBN 13: 978-0-415-95359-7 (hbk)

Visit the Taylor & Francis Web site at
http://www.taylorandfrancis.com

and the Routledge Web site at
http://www.routledgementalhealth.com

Contents

Series Editor's Foreword

The headline "Stress Disorder Linked to Soldiers' Ill Health" in the May 22, 2006 feature story of the *USA Today* Health Section by Marilyn Elias illustrates the contribution of *MindBody Medicine*, the newest book in the Routledge Psychosocial Stress Book Series. The article reports on a major government study of 3000 American combatants returning from the war in Iraq. Among other things, the study concluded that those with symptoms of post-traumatic stress disorder compared to those without these symptoms were in worse physical health, suffered more pain, and were more likely to miss work.

The study (Hoge et al., 2006) indicated that primary care doctors are hearing more physical complaints as the war continues and an increase in the number suffering (often-undiagnosed) from stress disorders, including but not limited to combat-related post-traumatic stress disorders. These complaints range from headaches to backaches and gastrointestinal complaints such as nausea and indigestion. Of course, the report noted that these complaints interfere with sleep, which in turn leads to low energy and efforts to use substances both to control the symptoms and to induce sleep, which in turn may lead to additional problems.

MindBody Medicine provides basic information and excellent guidance to physicians and other professionals working with veterans and others whose stress may manifest in such physical complaints as noted in the *USA Today* article. The multidisciplinary and interdisciplinary flavor of this book, so necessary for a seminal text on MindBody medicine, is due to the extraordinary qualifications and background of its authors.

Dr. Leo Rotan is director of Psychiatry/MindBody Medicine in the Family Practice Residency Program at Tallahassee Memorial Health Care and associate professor of medicine at the Florida State University School of Medicine in Tallahassee. Leo Rotan's education is varied; he earned an undergraduate degree in philosophy, master's degree in psychiatric social work, and doctoral degree in psychology with a dissertation on self-talk among male myocardial infarction patients. He has completed a long list of advanced training to improve his effectiveness as a practitioner. This includes advanced training in hypnosis, medical hypnosis, EMDR (eye movement desensitization and reprocessing), TFT (thought field therapy), MindBody medicine, spirituality and healing, psychoneuroimmunology, an American Psychosomatic Society update on research in psychosomatic illness, and attending four separate programs at Harvard University in alternative medicine and their program on MindBody medicine. He created and taught the first seminar in MindBody medicine at Florida State

University. He is a two-time winner of the Teacher of the Year award at the Family Medicine Residency Program. He is a Fellow of and board certified by the American College of Advanced Practice Psychologists.

Dr. Ospina-Kammerer is an adjunct professor in the Florida State University College of Social Work in Tallahassee; she studied under my supervision at Florida State University, including several years as a supervisor in my trauma clinic. She earned general nursing, psychiatric nursing, and teaching degrees in Europe before coming to the United States. In the U.S., she earned degrees in nursing, health education, social work, and marriage and family therapy. Her advanced training is in hypnosis, EMDR, TFT, MindBody medicine, spirituality and healing, and psychoneuroimmunology. Her various publications have been on stress-related MindBody health treatments. Since 1998, she has divided her time and teaching between Florida State University's College of Social Work and Austria's universities in Graz (Medizinische Universitaet Graz) and Innsbruck (UMIT–Private Universitaet fuer Gesundheitswissenschaften, Medizinische Informatik und Technik).

Dr. Ospina-Kammerer teaches and lectures at various universities throughout Europe in MindBody health, general mental health, general and psychiatric nursing, public health, crisis intervention, communication, and self-care. She has received numerous higher education teaching awards; she was awarded a Webstar for outstanding online, Web-based, and distance teaching for online blackboard courses throughout the United States; received awards for community service; and was awarded Diplomate of the American Psychotherapy Association (DAPA) status. She has an interesting background of working experience from Europe, England, South America, and the United States. She is also an international certified volunteer with hospice and a crisis intervention worker with Green Cross (disaster response) at my Traumatology Institute at Florida State University. She first met Dr. Rotan when she was a student of his at Florida State University. She worked as adjunct faculty in community medicine at the Tallahassee Memorial Health Care–Family Practice Residency Program.

Rotan and Ospina-Kammerer point out the importance of the psychosocial phenomena affecting our health, especially through the stress mechanism. Although stress and distress are often the *sine qua non* in most MindBody health and illness issues, the authors illustrate how stress is mediated by such factors as perceived social support, anger, forgiveness, anxiety, depression, and optimism. Their book helps the reader better appreciate the MindBody connection and how MindBody medicine can help modify behavior and attitudes, leading to better health.

Throughout this book, Rotan and Ospina-Kammerer discuss the interrelationships between a wide variety of diseases and other health problems and the activities of the mind that seem to influence these interactions. They note that, "Our thoughts (e.g., mental activities such as perception, belief, memory) play a powerful role in distress (e.g., perceiving and believing you are in great danger and being unable to escape may bring about a physical stress reaction even though there is no real objective danger)."

But one of the most important contributions of this book, and in line with the contributions of the other books in this series, is its focus on treatment: doing something and not just discussing the research and theory of the MindBody connection. Indeed, since the first book in the series on stress disorders among Vietnam veterans (1978), the series books have made contributions to the field not only through research and theory, but also through new and innovative ways of assessing and treating those affected by psychosocial stress. What sets this book apart from others in the series, however, is that *MindBody Medicine* provides a large array of techniques that can be used not only by practitioners but also by patients themselves. The dynamics of these techniques are further developed by consideration of mental activities, energy systems, and the psychosocial phenomena that all relate to the workings of MindBody medicine.

This book will be extremely useful for professors and students and working practitioners for expanding their appreciation for and application of MindBody medicine. It also is a practical handbook for the general public who wish to utilize powerful treatment and stress management procedures to improve their own health.

The series is dedicated to expanding the limits of what we know about the costs and benefits of psychosocial stress and how to use this knowledge to transform stress from a stumbling block into a stepping stone. *MindBody Medicine* is a giant stepping stone for patients and their practitioners who want to gain more control over the MindBody connection.

Charles R. Figley, Editor
Routledge Psychosocial Stress Book Series
Florida State University Traumatology Institute
Tallahassee, Florida

Preface

The patient[1] is deep in a hypnotic trance. This is apparent by her deep breathing, flatness of facial muscles, and calm expression. Through Dr. Rotan's coaching, she has trained herself to attain this state by self-hypnosis. In this, the third session, the patient has learned to control her migraine headaches without the use of medication. This is an example of MindBody medicine.

At a hospital in Cleveland, Ohio, children are taught to manage pain caused by their treatment. They use visual imagery to put themselves in a happy, comfortable state. They report feeling better and request fewer pain medications. This also is an example of MindBody medicine.

A 70-year-old hypertensive male patient was taught a meditation-relaxation technique, which he practiced daily for 20 minutes. After 3 days of practice, his systolic blood pressure was reduced by 12 points and his diastolic pressure by 8 points. This trend has remained consistent for the past 3 weeks of daily practice. This application of meditation to influence physical health is yet another example of MindBody medicine.

Perhaps you have read or heard reports of people meditating to lower their stress or using visual imagery to "see" their white blood cells eating invading germs. These are examples of MindBody medicine as well.

The next time you have the misfortune of stubbing your toe, hitting your thumb with the hammer, or scraping yourself when you fall, employ this simple MindBody intervention and discover how it works. (Remember, like any new skill, you may need to practice this several times.) Take a deep breath and visualize a favorite healing color. Then, let yourself feel the pain as you simultaneously visualize your color going into the injured and painful area. Imagine (i.e., see and feel) the color pushing out the pain and soreness and filling the area with healing light. Practice this technique and you will be surprised at how well this example of MindBody medicine works.

In this book, we help you explore the thought and science behind MindBody medicine. To aid in your exploration, we answer two questions: What is the mind? and What is MindBody medicine?

First, we define *mind*. We understand the mind to be the energy within ourselves that has the capability of performing cognitive functions. In humans, the mind is the energy channeled by the brain. We use the brain (an anatomical tool) to govern this energy. For further definitions, consult Appendix A.

As for MindBody medicine, we offer two definitions. The first comes from the National Institutes of Health (NIH). The second is from our own thoughts and experience. Before considering these definitions, take a moment to reflect and write your own definition. This is your first invitation to work in your book.

I define *MindBody medicine* as

____

____

Now, discover how your definition compares with the definition from the NIH and our definition.

According to the NIH, "Mind-body medicine focuses on the interactions among the brain, mind, body, and behavior, and the powerful ways in which emotional, mental, social, spiritual, and behavioral factors can directly affect health" and further, "Mind-body medicine typically focuses on intervention strategies that are thought to promote health, such as relaxation, hypnosis, visual imagery, meditation, yoga, biofeedback, tai chi, qugong, cognitive-behavioral therapies, group support, autogenic training, spirituality and prayer" (Complementary Alternative Medicine Web site, nccam.nih.gov 2005).

We offer an alternate definition: MindBody medicine is the study of how mental activities (e.g., beliefs) influence health and how using mental interventions (e.g., hypnosis) can change the content of these mental activities by either reducing stress or affecting cognitions or emotions to improve health.

However it is defined, MindBody medicine is becoming increasingly popular. The fact of this popularity is one reason why we have chosen to present a book that treats what we consider basic ideas in this area. We intend for this approach to serve as a beginning guide in an area that will change and grow. We hope to stimulate and challenge your thinking by including exercises at the end of each chapter. We hope to assist you in discovering, organizing, and acquiring knowledge about what is currently known in the scientific community about MindBody medicine.

Keep in mind that the science of MindBody medicine is in its infancy and recall that the first step in the scientific method is observation. Much of what you will read about MindBody medicine is still in the observation stage. Many claims have yet to be tested with true experimental design; however, this does not mean these claims are not true. It simply means that there is as yet insufficient scientific evidence of their validity.

We encourage you to be open, yet critical in your thinking. Like many nascent areas of scientific study, our inability to explain or understand how something works does not negate its reality. (For example, if you would have tried to explain the concept of the computer or telephone 200 years ago, you would have likely been met with disbelief.)

Please appreciate that what we present in this book is the beginning knowledge of something we will know more about as time goes on. You are likely to discover that some material we present now may become outdated, and you may feel frustrated that we have not gone into depth regarding how to employ specific interventions or given you magical mental healing skills. While this frustration is understandable, we hope it will motivate you to go to the next level and study the specific interventions you feel inclined to use. This can be best done by classes, conferences, and supervision with someone who possesses these skills. So, again, we stress the need to keep an open mind, yet a critical and inquisitive mind in your study of MindBody medicine.

Be encouraged by this observation by Kenneth Pelletier, PhD, MD: "Of all the complementary alternative therapies, mind/body-medicine is supported by the greatest body of scientific research for the greatest number of people." (Pelletier, 2002, p.13)

Introduction and Overview

Health and illness are often associated with our behavior, our emotions, and our thoughts (National Institutes of Health, 1992). For example, many cancers are associated with behaviors such as smoking. An emotion such as anger has been associated with coronary problems (Chang, 2002), and our thoughts play a powerful role in distress (e.g., perceiving and believing you are in great danger and cannot escape may bring about a physical stress reaction even though there is no real objective danger, etc.). Distress is associated with many illnesses (McEwen, 1993).

In MindBody medicine, we study interventions in order to change or strengthen mental activities, emotions, and behaviors related to health. MindBody medicine is focused on the interaction of mind and body. Becoming acquainted with these interventions and interactions is the purpose of this book. Below is a listing of topics to be studied and the approach that will be employed in presenting them.

TOPICS

Recall our definition of MindBody medicine: MindBody medicine is the study of how mental activities (e.g., beliefs) influence health and the utilization of MindBody interventions (e.g., hypnosis) to mediate these mental activities to produce healing and enrich health.

Taking this definition as our guide, we have divided the book into various topics (chapters). It is our intention that each topic will relate to the definition, either in part or as a whole, so at the end of your study you not only will have a deeper appreciation for what MindBody medicine is but also will have more confidence in understanding how MindBody medicine might be applied.

We have found in our teaching that most people who are interested in studying MindBody medicine prefer to begin their study with a look at the various techniques and interventions employed in the area of MindBody medicine. Thus, we start by helping you appreciate the variety of interventions at the disposal of a professional practicing MindBody medicine (Chapter 1).

We next share ideas about the mental activities that relate to these interventions, influence our state of well-being, and play a significant role in understanding MindBody medicine (Chapter 2).

Chapter 3 provides an overview of energy systems, an area that we believe will play a more significant role in understanding the mechanisms of MindBody medicine as research is better developed.

Then, you will attain a deeper understanding of the role of support, stress, and emotions—all factors related to our mental activity and overall health (Chapter 4).

Two important factors that need to be understood by professionals practicing MindBody medicine are stress and the physical systems thought to be most significant in MindBody interactions. Thus, we devote Chapter 5 (as well as Appendix C) to further development of ideas on stress and Chapter 6 to those key physical systems.

Chapters 1–5 supply good knowledge, but how to best apply it? We develop your understanding of applying MindBody medicine by presenting important questions to be answered before applying your knowledge (Chapter 6).

We further help you in understanding the application of this material by offering several examples of how this information has been applied to real cases. These examples are presented in Chapters 7 and 8.

In Chapter 9, we share some considerations of the ideas and interests of today's health care consumer, especially a look at employing MindBody medicine to enrich health rather than "cure" illness.

Finally, in Chapter 10, we offer some thoughts on the future direction of MindBody medicine.

APPROACH

As noted, the material in this book is presented in a workbook format. This means that each chapter helps you focus on the goals and objectives of that chapter. Following the goals and objectives, you will find a summary sharing of the basic information from the best research in MindBody medicine available up to 2006. Then, you have an opportunity to reinforce your learning by completing the exercises found at the end of each chapter.

In this rapidly growing field, new information develops in ways that make earlier hypotheses obsolete. Consequently, we suggest that you use the exercises as a review tool. In reviewing them periodically, you will give yourself an opportunity to update your knowledge since your old answers will change but the questions and guidelines in the exercises will remain useful. The approach presented here is a model to help you keep abreast of developments in the area of MindBody medicine.

After teaching graduate students for over 25 years, we also feel that if you are guided to investigate on your own, the information from your own effort will help you to realize much more from your investment of time and work. Each topic (each chapter treats a different topic) is organized in the following manner:

A. **Goals.** General information you wish to understand by working through the chapter.
B. **Learning objectives.** Specific things you will learn.
C. **Information guide.** Basic data to help you understand the subject.
D. **Readings.** Suggested literature for achieving your objectives.
E. **Exercises.** Suggestions to help you achieve your objectives.

By working through each chapter, you will develop your individual focus and interest while reinforcing the material you study. This guide may be used in a class, as part of continuing professional education, or to fulfill a personal interest to learn more about the exciting field of Mind-Body medicine. Although each chapter builds on the preceding one, you may approach them in any way that interests you. As you work through the guide, keep in mind your personal interests and general goals for developing a deeper understanding of MindBody medicine. In fact, it is recommended that you list those interests and goals before you begin.

My personal goals for studying MindBody medicine are:

____

____

____

____

____

As you work through each chapter you will see how much you learn.

Note that the journal *Advances in Mind-Body Medicine* (InnoVision Communications, e-mail: sladvances@aol.com) is a primary journal in this field. In general, we recommend you familiarize yourself with it and consider it recommended reading for each chapter.

For further thoughts on defining MindBody medicine, you might wish to consult the sources in the reading list.

SUGGESTED READING

Allison, N. (Ed.). (1999). *The Complete Body, Mind, and Spirit.* Chicago: Keats. [An excellent sourcebook for all areas of nontraditional healing.]

Astin, J. (2000). The efficacy of distant healing: A systematic review of randomized trials. *American Internal Medicine, 132,* 903–910. [Interesting review that might encourage further discussions on this topic.]

Astin, J.A., et al. (2003). Mind-Body medicine: State of science, implications for practice. *Journal of the American Board of Family Practice.* March, 16: 131–147 [This is an important information source for family practice physicians.]

Chang, P. (2002). Angry personality increases heart risk five-fold. *Archives of Internal Medicine, 162,* 901–906. [A well-done presentation on the importance of psychosocial issues such as anger.]

Davidson, K., et al. (2003). Evidence-based behavioral medicine: What is it and how do we achieve it? *Annals of Behavioral Medicine, 26,* 161–171.

Dreher, H. (1993). Mind body research and its detractors. *Advances, 9,* 59–62.

Goleman, D. (Ed.). (1993). *Mind Body Medicine.* Yonkers, New York: Consumer Reports Books. [This is an excellent sourcebook for obtaining a grasp of the entire area of MindBody medicine. The contributors use ample examples and understandable language and offer clear guidelines for practice. Goleman's book is a classic in MindBody medicine.]

McEwen, J. (1993). Stress and the individual mechanisms leading to disease. *Archives of Internal Medicine, 153,* 2093–2101. [In today's world of stress, this is important reading for each individual who wants to do everything possible to reduce and prevent stress.]

National Institutes of Health. (1992). *Alternative Medicine: Expanding Medical Horizons.* Washington, DC: U.S. Government Printing Office. [This report provides information important for practitioners and students at all levels of higher education.]

Pelletier, K. (2002). Mind as healer, mind as slayer: Mind Body medicine comes of age. *Advances, 18,* 4–13. [This is a very practical guide for understanding the power of the mind as healer.]

Sierpina, V. (2001). *Integrative Health Care: Complementary and Alternative Therapies for the Whole Person.* Philadelphia: F.A. Davis & Co.

1

MindBody Interventions

We are going to begin with an overview of the most researched MindBody interventions. These interventions are the tools for enhancing health by helping to strengthen or change mental activities and the behaviors and emotions those activities influence. This is an overview to introduce you to interventions that work and offer promise for extensive application in health. This is not meant to be complete. As you read and study MindBody medicine, you will discover more references and examples.

We offer a definition of the intervention, a short discussion to clarify the definition, examples of areas in which the intervention is thought to be successfully applied, examples of cases in which the intervention was employed, and a list of Suggested Reading. (For clarity, we include the Suggested Reading after the individual presentation of the intervention rather than at the chapter's end.) Note that some interventions can be learned for self-help; we include instructions to guide you in these.

The lists of interventions that follow are organized according to those that at this time have been more thoroughly researched to those that have been less so.

A. GOALS

1. To become familiar with various MindBody interventions.
2. To consider practical applications of MindBody interventions.

B. LEARNING OBJECTIVES

After working through this chapter, you should be able to

1. List the currently accepted MindBody interventions.
2. Match interventions to appropriate illness, medical procedures, or body systems.
3. Match illness to appropriate interventions.

C. INFORMATION GUIDE

MindBody Definitions

In your study of MindBody medicine, you will discover a variety of definitions. You will need to decide which definition makes the most sense to you in your work. It is likely that as more research occurs and you have more experience, your definition might change. Here, we state the "official" definition—that of the National Institutes of Health's National Center for Complementary and Alternative Medicine (NCCAM)—and then one that we find more workable from our work, research, and teaching of MindBody medicine.

NCCAM's definition is as follows:

> MindBody Medicine focuses on the interactions among the brain, mind, body, and behavior, and the powerful ways in which emotional, mental, social, spiritual, and behavioral factors can directly affect health. … MindBody Medicine typically focuses on intervention strategies that are thought to promote health, such as relaxation, hypnosis, visual imagery, meditation, yoga, biofeedback, tai chi, qigong, cognitive-behavioral therapies, group support, autogenic training, spirituality and prayer. (NCCAM, nccam.nih.gov, 2005)

From our teaching, practice, and research we are offering a somewhat different definition. We do not take a position that NCCAM is incorrect but rather that, in the current state of the science, there is still room for differences and refinement. Our definition is as follows:

> MindBody Medicine is the study of how mental activities influence health and how using mental interventions can change the content of these mental activities by either reducing stress or affecting cognitions or emotions in order to improve health. We define *mental activities* as the processes initiated by the mind (e.g., perceiving, imagining, and remembering). We discuss these at length in Chapter 2.

MINDBODY INTERVENTIONS

MindBody interventions are structured mental interventions (e.g., imagery) which employ primarily mental activities (e.g., perception) to enhance health.

The following section containing MindBody interventions is a basic introduction and overview. The current scientific knowledge about these interventions varies. For some (e.g., meditation, hypnosis) there is solid evidence of their effectiveness. For others (e.g., prayer, humor), the evidence is less so and in some cases there is debate regarding the quality of the research. Again, we remind you that just because an intervention is not yet fully "proven" by the scientific method does not mean that it is incorrect. This is also true if we cannot fully explain how the intervention might work. In answer to the legitimate question: Why include those interventions with questionable research behind them? We chose to include these because they are supported by a large enough representation of writers, institutions, or practitioners to warrant your awareness.

You will notice that our list of MindBody interventions is slightly different from the NCCAM. We include energy focus healing, expressive art, humor, poetry, expressive writing, and positive self-talk. These are included because they seem to meet the criteria of "structured mental interventions that employ primarily mental activities."

In energy focus healing, we look at those systems that rely on the healer (or patient) to employ mental activities to invoke or focus energy to an area of the body that requires attention. Expressive art seems to require active employment of mental activity such as memory and concentration, as does expressive writing. Humor certainly employs such things as cognitive constructing, imagination, and memory. Poetry seems by its definition to utilize the mind's ability to create, to imagine, and to remember (all mental activities).

WHAT IS MINDBODY, WHAT IS NOT?

In our review of the literature, we found confusion regarding just which interventions should be considered MindBody and which should not. In part, this confusion is because almost any human intervention is in some way associated with mental activity. So, in your critical study of MindBody medicine, remember that MindBody interventions are characterized by employing mental activities as the *primary* instrument by either the patient or practitioner.

In a different category are interventions, which though beneficial to the mind and body are primarily physical rather than primarily mental in application. These physical interventions are intentionally used to bring about a positive mental state such as relaxation or emotional release which, in turn, can benefit the body. In this category, we would include massage therapy, tai chi, qigong, exercise, and dance therapy.

In conclusion, the distinction between these two categories lies in the employment of mental activities as the primary tool of intervention.

1. Imagery

Definition. *Imagery* is a mental representation of a sensation either evoked or received.

Discussion. The use of imagination and hence imagery seems to be a part of being human. How often have you caught yourself daydreaming or plotting out a course of action using mental pictures? This type of creative activity can be applied to health. We are obtaining increased evidence that many people can, through imagination, effect the physiology of their bodies (Rossman, 1993). In the MindBody intervention of imagery, patients are helped to create pictures, memories, sounds, tactile sensation, and, yes, even smells. These images can be employed in many creative ways that suit the needs of the one using them. They are utilized to diagnose illnesses such as with a visual body scan. Many times through pictures patients learn to calm the tension in their muscles, lower their blood pressure, and create images of successful healing. Sometimes, these images are enhanced with hypnosis, and sometimes just using a relaxed state is sufficient. It is important to use images that are comfortable, not distressing, and that are suited to the interest of the one using them. Finally, in working with imagery to heal, the focus can be twofold. One focus may be on employing an image of the actual healing (e.g., a bone mending). The other may be to employ an image of the outcome of the healing (e.g., the use of the bone, such as in running).

Some Areas of Application

Asthma

Reduces episodes, reduces the use of medication, improves pulmonary function, and reduces specific immunoglobulin E responses (Castes et al., 1999).

Eating Disorders

Reduces binges and vomiting and improvement in self-concept (Esplen et al., 1998).

Immune System

Increases lymphocyte count and enhancement of natural killer cell function (Kiecolt-Glaser et al., 1985).

Shrinks cancer tumors (Dossey, 1999).

Changes individual lymphocyte count (Achterberg & Rider, 1993).

Medical Procedures

Alleviates nausea and vomiting in chemotherapy (Meyers & Mark, 1995; Brigham, 1990).

Prepares for surgery (Davis, 2002; Dreher, 1998).

Postsurgical recovery: lowers pain medication needs and decreases time to recovery (Lambert, 1996; Tusek, 1997).

Improves response to chemotherapy and improvement in self-image (Walker et al., 1999).

PAIN MANAGEMENT

Reduces or eliminates the sensation of pain (Kwekkenboom et al., 1998; Melzak, 1990; Meyers & Mark, 1995; Rossman, 1993, 1998; Syrjala et al., 1995).

Increases comfort in breast cancer treatment (Dolaba & Fox, 1999; Richardson et al., 1997).

Illustrations

A patient with an immune-compromising disease is assisted with guided imagery of her natural killer cells becoming strong and attacking the invading organism. She could picture her cells in any fashion that would seem powerful to her (e.g., white knights killing the invading cells). [Note that a more auditory patient might hear her cells rather than see them.] This would be done with input from the patient regarding which images appeal to her. She may spend 20 minutes a day doing this exercise in a relaxed state.

Ms. A was terrified of her upcoming chemotherapy. She was interested in any approach that might help. Since she was an accomplished musician, she was able to hear and "see" sounds; that is, she could use her imagination to bring these musical notes into her auditory and visual domains. This talent was utilized by training her in an imaging technique in which she would start a "mental" musical event while in the waiting area for her chemotherapy. She carried this out throughout her treatment. Her reports of her experience indicated that this method helped her be totally relaxed and surprisingly free of discomfort.

Mr. L. experienced difficulties falling asleep. He pictured himself laying in a hammock and feeling a light wind moving his hammock gently. He would use this technique every night, and he could easily fall asleep.

Ms. G., who is underweight, wanted to gain a few additional pounds by using imagery. Ms. G. pictured herself in one of her favorite dresses that she could not wear anymore because it was too large for her. She practiced this exercise twice a day by looking at a picture of her wearing her favorite dress. Ms. G. was also eating more sensibly and putting on a few additional pounds.

Mr. J., a high-school student, is ridiculed by his peers because he was overweight. Mr. J. pictured himself in one of his favorite sportswear outfits that he could not wear anymore because it was too small for him. He practiced this exercise twice a day by looking at a picture of himself from a previous sports tournament. Mr. J. also followed a sensible diet to help him to stay healthy.

SUGGESTED READING

Achterberg, J., & Rider, M.S. (1993). The effects of music mediated imagery on neutrophils and lymphocytes. *Biofeedback and Self Regulation, 14,* 247–257. [Achterberg is a classical researcher in the entire area of MindBody medicine, especially imagery. This article is a good example of her interest and work.]

Brigham, D.D. (1990). *The Use of Imagery in a Multimodal Psycho-Neuro-Immunology Program for Cancer and Other Chronic Diseases.* New York: Plenum Press.

Castes, M., Hagel, I., et al. (1999). Immunologic changes associated with clinical improvement of asthmatic children subjected to psychosocial intervention. *Brain, Behavior and Immunity, 13,* 1–13.

Davis, D. (2002, November 9–10). *Guided imagery prepares patients for surgery while reducing charges for care: A health plan sponsored program.* Report from Blue Shield of California presented at the Society of Clinical and Experimental Hypnosis 53rd annual scientific program, Boston. [This report is significant in that it outlines the approach of a major insurance provider in paying for a MindBody intervention.]

Dolaba, K., & Fox, C. (1999). The effects of guided imagery on comfort of women with early stage breast cancer undergoing radiation therapy. *Oncology Nursing Forum, 26,* 67–72.

Dossey, L. (1999). *Reinventing Medicine.* San Francisco: Harper. [Dossey comes from a different background and belief about the area of MindBody medicine. As he became more aware of the significant interaction of the mind and body, he became active in writing provocative and informative information that is both useful and inspirational.]

Dreher, H. (1998). Mind-Body interventions for surgery: Evidence and exigency. *Advances, 14,* 207–222.

Esplen, M.J., et al. (1998). A randomized controlled trial of guided imagery in bulimia nervosa. *Psychological Medicine, 28,* 1347–1357.

Kiecolt-Glaser, J., et al. (1985). Psycho-social enhancement of immunocompetence in a geriatric population. *Health Psychology, 4,* 25–29.

Kwekkenboom, K., et al. (1998). Imaging ability and effective use of guided imagery. *Research in Nurse Health, 21,* 189–198.

Lambert, S.A. (1996). The effects of hypnosis/guided imagery on the post operative course of children. *Journal of Developmental Behavioral Pediatrics,* 17, 307–10.

Melzak, R. (1990). The tragedy of needless pain. *Scientific American, 262,* 27–33. [Melzak is a classic researcher in the area of pain, and this article serves as a needed reference for approaches such as imagery.]

Meyers, T.J., & Mark, M.M. (1995). Effects of psychosocial interventions on adult cancer patients. A meta-analysis of randomized experiments. *Health Psychology, 14,* 101–108. [An excellent article to bring you up to 1995 with the best research.]

Richardson, M.A., et al. (1997). Coping, life attitudes, and immune response to imagery and group support after breast cancer treatment. *Alternative Therapies in Health and Medicine, 3,* 62–70.

Rossman, M. (1993). Imagery: Learning to use the mind's eye. In D. Goleman (Ed.), *Mind Body Medicine.* (pp. 291–300). Yonkers, NY: Consumer Reports Books. [Dr. Rossman is one of the foremost thinkers and researchers in the application of imagery to healing. Because of the quality of his work, we even include one as old as 1989.]

Rossman, M. (1989). *Healing Yourself: A Step-by-Step Program for Better Health Through Imagery.* New York: Pocket Books.

Syrjala, K.L., et al. (1995). Relaxation and imagery and cognitive-behavioral training reduce pain during cancer treatment: A controlled clinical trial. *Pain, 63,* 189–198.

Tusek, D., Church, J., et al. (1997). Guided imagery. A significant advance in the care of patients undergoing elective colorectal surgery. *Diseases of the Colon and Rectum, 40,* 172–178.

Walker, L.G., et al. (1999). Psychological, clinical and pathological effects of relaxation training and guided imagery during primary chemotherapy. *British Journal of Cancer, 80,* 262–268.

Instructions for Imagery

Example 1

1. Put your self in a quiet safe place.
2. Get in a comfortable position.
3. Take five slow deep breaths (hold each breath for 5 seconds before exhaling).
4. Picture a color or imagine a sound that appeals to you and is comfortable for you.
5. Gently focus this color/sound to the area in your body that needs healing.
6. See and hear this color/sound changing that area in some way (e.g., pushing out the pain and filling the area with the color/sound; melting away a tumor; stopping blood flow, enhancing blood flow).

Example 2

In this approach, you focus your imaging on a final result you desire instead of the disease, pain or injury. Take a broken leg as an example. Instead of focusing healing energy on mending a leg, you focus on the final result, such as the leg functioning as a healed leg should. That is, you imagine yourself walking, running, dancing, and so on.

2. Meditation

Definition. *Meditation* involves a focused state of calmness and detached awareness.

Discussion. Meditation is an ancient practice of putting oneself (or allowing oneself to go) into a state of focused, calm awareness. Note that meditation is not daydreaming or even imagery. It is not an altered state like hypnosis. The hallmark of meditation is being in the present moment.

The approach of meditation has been employed in a variety of settings and contexts. It has ancient roots in religion as well as in the training of warriors. These diverse environments are primarily because of the value meditation offers as a help to focusing and awareness. This help is likely the value meditation offers for application to health issues.

Meditation helps you become relaxed (it brings about a physiological response called the relaxation response (RR), which is considered separately in this chapter). The other "power" in meditation is that it is a practice in letting go of thought and feeling and placing yourself in the here and now. In doing this, the mediator becomes able to let go of anxieties and concerns about the past and future. This calm focus and ability to let go may be one of the variables of the healing power of meditation.

Generally, there are two broad areas of meditation: concentration and mindfulness. In both approaches, remember that meditation is a state of focused, calm awareness.

Concentration

In concentration, your attention is focused and controlled (concentrated) on one thing, such as the repetition of a word or phrase (this could be a short prayer or a simple positive self-statement such as "peace," "calm"). In some traditions, this word or phrase may be referred to as a *mantra*. Some mediators preferred to use a sound or simply count their breaths. As you concentrate on the object (i.e., a word or your breathing), you let go of all other thoughts/ideas, keeping your attention and focus simply in the here and now. Much research in health has been carried out employing a form of this meditation called transcendental meditation.

Mindfulness

Mindfulness meditation is very similar to concentration. In fact, many mediators will often start their mindfulness meditation with a short period of concentration. In mindfulness, you simply note any thoughts or feelings as they occur. You observe them intentionally without judgment moment by moment, allowing them to gently float away from you. Be aware of your feelings and reactions that occur. Note your feelings, allow them to be part of your here and now but do not spend time or effort thinking about them. Let them also float away. Much research utilizing mindfulness meditation has been carried out and published by Jan Kabatt-Zinn at the University of Massachusetts School of Medicine.

This awareness, acceptance, and allowing yourself to let go will likely be seen as an important variable in meditation's healing power. Often in the practice of psychotherapy, we discover that much suffering happens because of an inability to recognize and acknowledge that painful experiences and feelings are part of our life situation, and by accepting them as such and letting them go rather than spending much effort in denying them or taking medication to rid ourselves of them we are able to live more healthfully. As therapists, we recognize that this acceptance and letting go is far from easy. Again, meditation can serve as the tool that helps us train to recognize, accept, and let go.

Some Areas of Application

Anxiety

Decreases anxiety (Brown, 2003; Miller, Fletcher, et al., 1995; NIH, 1999; Schneider & Staggters, 2005; Speca, 2000).

Cardiovascular

Blood vessel blockage: prevents heart attack or stroke (Castillo-Richmond & Schneider, 2002).

Reduces cholesterol levels (NIH, 1999).

Reduces high blood pressure (Alexander, 1996; Barnes, 2000, 2003; NIH, 1999; Schneider, 1995).

Insomnia

Improves sleep patterns (NIH, 1999).

Immune System

Increases antibody titers to influenza vaccine (Davidson et al., 2003).

Pain Management

Reduces chronic pain (Caudill et al., 1991; Kabat-Zinn, 1986).

Mood

Decreases depression (Brown, 2003; Segal, 2001 Teastate, 2002).

Fewer relapses with mindfulness meditation and cognitive group therapy than control group (Santorelli, 1999).

Long-term improvement in mood (Shapiro et al., 2001).

Skin

Enhances improvement in psoriasis (mindfulness) (Kabat-Zinn, 2000; Polenghi et al., 1994).

Stress

Lowers stress and coping with stress and burnout (Miller et al., 1995; Ospina-Kammerer & Dixon, 2001).

Illustrations

A patient with chronic hypertension and pain is instructed in meditation. After 3 weeks of 20 minutes of daily practice of a simple meditation technique (counting inhalations and exhalations to ten and then repeating the count for the full 20 minutes), she reported an improvement in her perception of pain. To the treating physician's surprise, her blood pressure was lowered from 150/90 to 138/80; these results have now lasted for a year, and she continues with her meditation.

Another example of meditation utilized a breathing technique, including the use of a phrase "let go," to reduce stress in family physician residents during stressful working hours in a emergency room (Ospina-Kammerer & Figley, 2003).

Kabat-Zinn (2000) described an approach he labeled the walking meditation (WM) as a simple way to reduce stress. Walking not only is a simple and healthy form of exercise, but also is a simple way of bringing awareness into a person's life. Kabat-Zinn suggests people should bring their attention to the actual experience of walking as they are doing it. In WM, you do not explore the surroundings as you walk but keep your eyes focused in front of you. If the mind wanders away, then the author suggests simply to bring it back and feel the sensations of walking. This same approach was presented in audiotape format by Goleman (1989), directed toward clients who may have difficulty remaining seated while attempting to achieve a level of calm or relaxation. The WM is an excellent stress-reducing method.

We use both concentration and mindfulness in our daily lives (two times a day for 20 minutes). This practice helps us remain more calmly in the here and now, concentrate more fully on our patients, and be less encumbered with the past or concerned about the future.

SUGGESTED READING

Alexander, C.N., Barnes, V., Schneider, R.H., (1996) A randomized controlled trial of stress reduction on cardiovascular and all cause mortality: results of 8 years and 15 years follow up. *Circulation 93*(9). 629.

Barnes, V. (1999). Acute effects of transcendental meditation on hemodynamic functioning in middle age adults. *Psychosomatic Medicine 61*, 525–531. [This is a good explanation of how meditation might fit into healing.]

Barnes, V. (2003). Impact of transcendental meditation on cardiovascular function at rest and during acute stress in adolescents with high normal blood pressure. *Journal of Psychosomatic Research, 51*, 597–605. [A very important reference for mental health care workers who work with clients who experience psychosomatic illness.]

Brown, K.W. (2003). The benefits of being present: Mindfulness and its role in psychological well-being. *Journal of Personal and Social Psychology, 84*, 822–848.

Castillo-Richmond & Schneider, R.H. (2002). Effects of stress reduction on carotid atherosclerosis in hypertensive African Americans. *Stroke, 31*, 568. [Reducing stress and preventing hypertension and stroke are important factors both discussed in this work.]

Caudill, M., et al. (1991). Decreased Clinic Use by chronic pain patients: response to behavioral medicine interventions. *Clinical Journal of Pain, 7*, 305–310 [This is important reading for health care workers in the medical field since more than 60% of patients visiting family physicians are experiencing chronic pain.]

Davidson, R.J., et al. (2003). Alterations in brain and immune function produced by mindfulness meditation. *Psychosomatic Medicine, 65*, 564–570.

Goleman, D. (1989). *Mind Body Medicine.* Yonkers, NY: Consumer Reports Books.

Kabat-Zinn, J. (1986). Four year follow up of meditation based program for the self-regulation of chronic pain. *Clinical Journal of Pain, 2*, 150–173.

Kabat-Zinn, J. (2000). Report of the annual Harvard Scientific Conference on Alternative Medicine. *Psychosomatic Medicine,* (1998) *60,* 625–632.

Kabat-Zinn, J., et al. (1998). Influence of a mindfulness meditation-based stress reduction intervention on rates of skin clearing in patients with moderate to severe psoriasis undergoing phototherapy, and photochemotherapy. *Psychosomatic Medicine, 60,* 625–632. [Kabat-Zinn has long researched and applied mindfulness meditation to a variety of medical and psychological conditions. Because of this, he should be on the reading list of any student of MindBody medicine.]

Miller, J., Fletcher, K., et al. (1995). Three year follow-up and clinical implications of a mindfulness meditation-based stress reduction intervention in the treatment of anxiety disorders. *General Hospital Psychiatry, 17,* 192–200. [The authors emphasized the importance of stress reduction in today's society through simple mindfulness meditation.]

National Institutes of Health. www.nih.gov. Retrieved October 12, 1999.

NIH Fields of Practice. (1999). National Institutes of Health Web site. [This will bring you up to date on the government position concerning approaches in MindBody medicine.]

Ospina-Kammerer, V. & Dixon, D.R. (2001). Coping with burnout: Family physicians and family social workers—what do they have in common? *Journal of Family Social Work, 5,* 85–93. [This article offers the practical tool of walking meditation that every person can find useful.]

Ospina-Kammerer, V., & Figley, C.R. (2003). An evaluation of the respiratory one method (ROM) in reducing emotional exhaustion among family physician residents. *International Journal of Emergency Mental Health, 5*(1), 29–32. [The respiratory one method is a practical application that every person may find not only personally helpful, but also useful when working with clients or patients. Ospina-Kammerer, one of the authors of this book, presents an example of applying meditation is a real environment.]

Polenghi, M.M., Molinari, E., Gala, C., Guzzi, R., Garutti, C., & Finzi, A.F. (1994). Experience with psoriasis in a psychosomatic dermatology clinic. *Acta Dermato-venereologica. Supplementum (Stockholm), 186,* 65–66.

Santorelli, S.F. (1999). *Heal Thyself, Lessons on Mindfulness in Medicine.* New York: Random House-Bell Tower.

Schneider, R.H., Staggters, F., et al. (1995). A randomized controlled trial of stress reduction for hypertension in older African Americans. *Hypertension, 26,* 820–827.

Segal, Z. (2000). *Mindfulness Based Cognitive Therapy for Depression.* New York: Guilford Press. [Segal elaborates on mindfulness and how it can be integrated into cognitive therapy to help people with anxiety and depression.]

Shapiro, S.L., et al. (2001). Meditation and positive psychology. In C. R. Snyder and S. Lopex (Eds.), Handbook of Positive Psychology. New York: Oxford University Press. pp. 632–634. [This is an excellent resource for every student of MindBody medicine.]

Speca, M. (2000). A randomized, waitlist controlled clinical trial: the effect of a mindfulness meditation based stress reduction program on mood and symptoms stress in cancer patients. *Psychosomatic Medicine, 62,* 613–622.

Teastate, J. D. (2002). Relapse-recurrence in major depression by mindfulness based cognitive therapy. *Journal of Consulting and Clinical Psychology, 68,* 615–623.

Instruction on an Approach to Meditation

- Secure a safe, quiet place with minimum disturbances.
- Sit in a comfortable but alert position.
- Close your eyes, hold them half open or focus them on a calm simple object (e.g., a candle, flower).
- Allow yourself to breath comfortably deep and slowly with slight holding of the breath on inhalation.
- Be aware of your breathing and any body sensations and adjust any uncomfortable position.
- Begin to count your breaths (one in, two out, three in, four out, etc., up to ten and repeat this process for the entire time).

As thoughts come, emotions arise, and distractions occur, just allow them to float away (do not think about them, try to work them out, or in any way give them attention).

Continue this process for up to 20 minutes and do it twice a day (much research has been done with meditation occurring for up to 45 minutes). Start slowly (5 minutes) and work up to longer sessions.

Remember that this is just one approach; meditation is not contemplation (i.e., you are not thinking about something and trying to work on it); meditation is not imagery; it is a state of focused awareness.

3. Psychotherapy

Definition. *Psychotherapy* involves focused interchanges (usually verbal) between a psychologically trained professional and a client. The purpose of this interchange is the client's well-being, either through the prevention or curing of a specific malfunction or the development of insight for personal enrichment.

Discussion. The basic ingredient in psychotherapy seems to us to be the interchange of information between a client or patient and a trained professional for the purposes listed in the definition. This exchange has taken on a variety of expressions. In part, this variety is accounted for because of the theoretical model on which the therapy is built. In simple terms, the wide umbrella of psychotherapy includes the classical analytical approach, the behavioral approach, and the humanistic approach. There can be found all types of permutations and expressions of these basic approaches throughout psychotherapy's history. In fact, we have found claims of as many as 240 different types of psychotherapy.

In our concern of applying psychotherapy to health, the most researched approach to date (2006) has been the cognitive-behavioral approach, followed by the interpersonal approach and with small nods to behavioral and psychoanalytically oriented approaches.

Psychotherapy's claim to a place as a MindBody intervention is strengthened by the research indicating that in psychotherapy there are measurable changes in brain anatomy and brain area involvement.

As we stated, most reported research has utilized cognitive-behavioral psychotherapy. In the following examples, we note which type of psychotherapy is reported as the intervention if other than a cognitive-behavioral approach.

Some Areas of Application

Anxiety

Psychotherapy decreases anxiety (Barlow, 1996).

Improves obsessive-compulsive disorders 70% (Schwartz, 1996).

Depression

Decreases faster and stays away longer than with medication alone, with cognitive therapy, or with interpersonal therapy (Antonuccio, 1998; Keller, 2000).

Psychotherapy as effective as medication (Depression Guideline Panel, 1993; Mayberg, 2003).

Psychotherapy as effective as medication in managing mild-to-moderate depression (Rupke, 2006).

Cognitive-behavioral psychotherapy as effective as light treatment in treating seasonal affective disorder (Rohan, 2004).

Note that many readings on "psychotherapy" offer effective treatment options for clients who suffer any type of anxiety or depression.

Hypertension

Reduces both systolic and diastolic pressure (Linden, 1994; Schneider, 1995).

Decreases levels of blood pressure (diastolic and mean arterial pressure), heart rate, and rate pressure product (Lawler et al., 2003).

Irritable Bowel Syndrome

Stabilizes condition: Decreases incidents and lowers the need for pain medication (Haymann-Monnikes, Arnold, Flound, et al., 2000; Read, 1999; Palson, 2006).

Psychotherapy equal to medication in effectiveness (Blanchard & Malamood, 1996).

Immune System

Improves management of herpes 2 virus with cognitive-behavioral therapy (Lutgendorf, 1997).

Medical Procedures

Psychologically prepares patient for breast reconstruction (Matheson, 1990).

Chronic Pain

Helps with pain management (Winterowed, Beck, et al., 2003).

Effective in modifying lower back pain (Van Talden et al., 2000).

Panic Disorders

Better than medication for long-term management of panic attacks (Barlow, 1996).

Sleep Disorders

Reduces insomnia (reduces time awake after sleep onset) (Jacob, 2004; Morin et al., 1999).

Increases the quality of sleep time (Smith & Perles, 2006).

Skin

Reduces or cures psoriasis (Grossbart, 1993).

Suicide

Cognitive therapy reduces the risk of suicide (Brown, 2005).

Illustrations

A patient with depression and intense headache with no apparent physical cause is helped through cognitive restructuring, free association, and reflective association to get in touch with her repressed anger toward an abusive father. Her awareness and ability to ventilate and process her feelings, change her cognitive labeling, tie information together, and accept herself and her limitations in an accepting and empathetic environment results in minimizing the depression and eliminating her headache.

A patient with psychosomatic disorder is learning breathing techniques and new coping skills in dealing with somatic symptoms. For a breathing technique, the patient inhales through the nose, exhales through the mouth, and uses the number 7 as a reminder to do it seven times in one setting and seven times a day.

Cognitive-behavioral therapy is used to lower stress in a patient with an immune disorder. As the patient learns to recognize, restructure his perceptions and self-talk in the empathetic environment of therapy, his reactions are changed. Thus, when formally stressful situations arise he has learned to clarify the situation, label it correctly, and apply skills to letting it go or applying a remedy. After five sessions, his disorder is under control.

SUGGESTED READING

Antonuccio, D. (1998). The coping with depression course: A behavioral treatment for depression. *Clinical Psychology, 51,* 3–5.

Barlow, D.H. (1996). Advances in psychosocial treatment of anxiety disorders. *Archives of General Psychiatry, 53,* 727–735. [Barlow is one of the foremost researchers in the field of anxiety. This and most of his work are important references in the field.]

Barlow, D. (2000). Cognitive behavioral therapy, imipramine, or their combination for panic disorders: A randomized controlled trial. *Journal of the American Medical Association, 283,* 2529–2536.

Blanchard, E., & Malamood, H.S. (1996). *Professional Psychology: Research and Practice.*

Brown, G. (2005). Cognitive therapy reduces suicide risk. *Journal of the American Medical Association, 294,* 563–70, 623–624. [This article is a good review of the application of this most-researched psychotherapy intervention.]

Cruess, S. (2000). Reduction in herpes simplex virus type 2 antibody titers after cognitive behavioral stress management and relationship with neuroendocrine function, relaxation skills, and social support in HIV positive men. *Psychosomatic Medicine, 62,* 828–837.

Grossbart, T. (1993). The skin matters of the flesh. In D. Goleman (Ed.), *Mind Body Medicine.* (pp. 145-160). Yonkers, NY: Consumer Reports Books

Haymamm-Monnikes, I., & Arnold, R. (2000). The combination of medical treatment plus multi-component behavioral therapy is superior to medical treatment alone in the therapy of irritable bowel syndrome. *American Journal of Gastroenterology, 95,* 981–944. [The authors offer hope by applying behavioral therapy aside medical treatment for clients who suffer irritable bowel syndrome.]

Jacob, G.D. (2004). Cognitive behavior therapy and pharmacotherapy for insomnia: A randomized control trial and direct comparison. *Archives of Internal Medicine, 164,* 1888–1896.

Keller, M.B. (2000). A comparison of nefrazodone, cognitive behavioral analysis system of psychotherapy, and their combination in the treatment of chronic depression. *New England Journal of Medicine, 342,* 1462–1470. [This article is important for mental health care workers and students in the mental health fields.]

Lawler, K.A., Younger, J.W., Piferi, R.L., Billington, E., Jobe, R, Edmondson, K., et al. (2003). A change of heart: Cardiovascular correlates of forgiveness in response to interpersonal conflict. *Journal of Behavior Medicine, 26,* 373–393. [The authors document the importance of forgiveness and the correlating factors with cardiovascular problems.]

Linden, W.C. (1994). Clinical effectiveness of non-drug treatment for hypertension. A meta-analysis. *Annuals of Behavioral Medicine, 16,* 35–45.

Lutgendorf, S.K., Michael, H.A., Gail, I., Klimas, N., Fletcher, M.N., & Schneiderman, N. (1997). Cognitive processing style, mood, and immune function following HIV seropositivity notification. *Cognitive Therapy and Research, 21*(2), 157–184

Matheson, G.D. (1990). Psychological preparation of the patient for breast reconstruction. *Annals of Plastic Surgery, 24,* 238–247.

Mayberg, H. (2003). *Archives of General Psychiatry, 61.*

Morin, C.M., et al. (1999). A randomized controlled trial of stress reduction for hypertension in older African Americans. *Hypertension, 6*, 820–827.
Palson, O. (2006). The nature of IBS and the need for a psychological approach. *International Journal of Clinical and Experimental Hypnosis, 54*, 1–5.
Read, N.W. (1999). Harnessing the patient's power. *Baillieres Best Practice and Research in Clinical Gastroenterology, 13*, 473–487.
Rohan, K. (2004). Seasonal affective disorders and psychotherapy. *Journal of Affective Disorders, 80*, 273–283.
Rupke, S., et al. (2006). Cognitive therapy for depression. *American Family Physician*, 73.
Schneider, R.H., et al. (1995). A randomized controlled trial of stress reduction for hypertension in older African Americans. *Hypertension, 26*, 820–827.
Schwartz, J.M., Stoessel, P.W., Baxter, Jr., L.R., Martin, K.M., & Phelps, M.E. (1996). Systematic changes in cerebral glucose metabolic rate after successful behavior modification treatment of obsessive-compulsive disorder. *Archives General Psychiatry, 53*, 109–113. [This is an excellent review and update on the power of good psychotherapy.]
Smith, M., & Perles, M. (2006). Who is a candidate for cognitive-behavioral therapy for insomnia? *Health Psychology, 25*, 15–19. [This is important reading for practitioners and clients who experience sleeping problems.]
Van Talden, M.W., et al. (2000). Analysis of research. *Spine, 26*, 270–281.
Winterowed, C., Beck, A., et al. (2003). *Cognitive Therapy With Chronic Pain Patients.* New York: Springer.

4. Hypnosis

Definition. *Hypnosis* is an altered state of consciousness with focused attention.

Discussion. Hypnosis is the skill to focus your attention in such a manner that it screens out unwanted stimuli. In employing hypnosis for health care, there is usually a trained hypnotherapist that assists (like a coach) the patient in achieving this level of attention, known as a *trance*. In our work with hypnosis, we often train the patient to use self-hypnosis and to learn to achieve this level of focus on their own. With this focusing, some people are able to be so attuned to suggestion they eliminate sensation such as pain and perceive imagined events as if they were real and in doing so influence the body to react. This is dramatically demonstrated in the ability to eliminate the sensation of pain, to move blood to various parts of the body, or to bring about a sympathetic nervous response. Although an ancient tool for health, hypnosis is currently under investigation by employing measuring instruments such as functional magnetic resonance imaging to learn about its dynamics (Raz, 2005).

Some Areas of Application

Anxiety

Reduces anxiety (Barlow, 1996).

Childbirth

Converts breech presentation (Mehl, 1994).

Dermatology

Hypnosis helps with a variety of skin conditions (Shenefelt, 2000).

Eating Disorders

Helps control bulimia, anorexia, and obesity (Barabasz, 1989).

Gastrointestinal Problems

Improves functional dyspepsia (Calvert, Houghton, Cooper, Morris, & Whorwell, 2002).

Immune System

Increases T and B cells (Ruzylasmith et al., 1995).

Irritable Bowel Syndrome

Improves irritable bowel syndrome (Blanchard, 1996; Gonsalkorale, Houghton, & Whorwell, 2000; Palsson, 2006; Palsson, Turner, Johnson, Burnett, & Whitehead, 2006; Whitehead, 2006).

Medical Procedures

Reduces need for sedating medication (Lang & Joyce, 1996).

Reduces/eliminates nausea from chemotherapy (Meyer, 1995).

Requires less analgesia and a reduction in hospital stay with surgical patients (Lang, Berotsh, & Fick, 2000).

Panic Disorders

As effective as medications in treating panic disorder and agoraphobia (Gallo, 1999).

More effective than medications for long-term durability (Barlow, 2000).

Pain

Reduces general pain (Liossi & Hatura, 2003; Raz, 2005).

Use for temporal mandibular disorder (NIH/OAM, 1998).

Treats pain from severe burns (Patterson, Adcock, & Bombardier, 1997).

Illustrations

A patient was referred to the first author because of terror of needles. The patient was trained in hypnosis to interpret the needle stick as a feathery tickle. She is now able to laugh as she has a needle injection or has blood drawn.

A patient who needed to undergo an imaging test that required her to be in a closed environment requested hypnosis to help with her anxiety. After two sessions, she learned to induce a trance and in this state learned to transport herself to a wonderful open area that she remembered as a child. She used this to stop her anxiety and was able undergo the needed test with ease.

SUGGESTED READING

Barlow, D.H. (1996). Advances in the psychosocial treatment of anxiety disorders. *Archives of General Psychiatry, 53*, 727–735.

Barlow, D. (2000).Cognitive behavioral therapy, imipramin or their combination for panic disorders: A randomized controlled trial *Journal of the American Medical Association, 283*, 2529–2536. [Barlow is a key researcher in the area of anxiety. His findings on this topic and hypnosis are significant to the entire field of health.]

Barabasz, M. (1989). Treatment of bulimia with hypnosis involving awareness and control in clients with high dissociative capacity. *International Journal* of *Psychosomatic Medicine, 36*, 104–108.

Bennet, H. (1986). Behavioral anesthesia. *Advances, 2*.

Blanchard, E.B., & Scharff, L. (2002). Psychosocial aspects of assessment and treatment of irritable bowel syndrome in adults and recurrent abdominal pain in children. *Journal of Consulting and Clinical Psychology, 70*, 725–738.

Calvert, E.L., Houghton, L.A., Cooper, P., Morris, J., & Whorwell, P.J. (2002). Long-term improvement in functional dyspepsia using hypnotherapy. *Gastroenterology, 123*, 1778–1785.

Gallo, F. (1999). *Innovations in Psychology*. Boca Raton, FL: CRC Press. [Gallo's work is an invaluable reference in the exciting area of the "manipulation of energy" to bring about change, particularly the approach of thought field therapy.]

Gonsalkorale, W.M., Houghton, L.A., & Whorwell, P.J. (2002). Hypnotherapy in irritable bowel syndrome: A large-scale audit of a clinical service with examination of factors influencing responsiveness. *American Journal of Gastroenterology, 97*, 954–961. [This article is a useful review of an important area, the value of hypnosis in treating an area that often is approached with medications only.]

Lang, D.V., Berotsh, E.G., & Fick, L.J. (2000). Adjunctive non-pharmacological analgesia for medical procedures. *Lancet, 355*, 1486–1490. [Hospital and outpatient surgery settings could not only help clients by reducing unnecessary pain, but also evaluate the economical factor of nonpharmacological analgesia for medical procedures.]

Lang, E.V., Joyce, J.S., Spiegal, D. (1996). Self hypnotic relaxation during interventional radiological procedures: effects on pain perception and intravenous drug use. *Journal of Clinical and Experimental Hypnosis 44*, 106–119.

Liossi, C., & Hatura, P. (2003). Clinical hypnosis in the alleviation of procedure related pain in pediatric oncology patients. *International Journal of Clinical and Experiential Hypnosis, 57,* 4–28. [This provides important information for health care professionals working with pediatric and oncology patients.]

Lutgendorf, S.K., Michael, H. A., Gail, I., Klimas, N., Fletcher, M.N., & Schneiderman, N. (1997). Cognitive processing style, mood, and immune function following HIV seropositivity notification. *Cognitive Therapy and Research, 21*(2), 157–184.

Menhl, L.E. (1994). Hypnosis and conversion of the breech to the vertex presentation. *Archives of Family Medicine, 3,* 881–887.

Meyers, T.J., & Mark, M.M. (1995). Effects of psychosocial interventions with adult cancer patients: A meta-analysis of randomized experiments. *Health Psychology, 14,* 101–108

NIH/OAM Consensus Report, Panel 5 (1998).

Palsson, O.S. (2006). Standardized hypnosis treatment for irritable syndrome: The North Carolina protocol. *The International Journal of Clinical and Experimental Hypnosis, 54,* 51–64.

Palsson, O.S., Turner, M.J., Johnson, D.A., Burnett, C.K., & Whitehead, W.E. (2002). Hypnosis treatment for severe irritable bowel syndrome—Investigation of mechanism and effects on symptoms. *Digestive Diseases and Sciences, 47,* 2605–2614. [Dr. Palsson has long been involved in research and practice in the area. This article presents an excellent update and overview of a clear application of MindBody medicine.]

Patterson, D.R., Adcock, R.J., & Bombardier, C.H. (1997). Factors predicting hypnotic analgesia in clinical burn pain. *The International Journal of Clinical and Experimental Hypnosis, 55,* 377–395.

Raz, A. (2005). Hypnotic suggestion reduces conflict in the human brain. *Proceedings of the National Academy of Sciences, 102,* 9978–9983. [This prestigious group's conclusions in this area is an important document for anyone interested in the field.]

Ruyylasmith, P., et al. (1995). Effects of hypnosis on the immune response: B-cells, T-cells, helper and suppressor cells. *American Journal of Clinical Hypnosis, 38,* 71–79.

Shenefelt, P.D. (2000). Hypnosis in dermatology. *Archives of Dermatology, 136,* 393–399. [Shenefelt's report will give you a valuable and empirical focus on this entire area of dermatology.]

Whitehead, W. (2006). Hypnosis for irritable bowel syndrome: The empirical evidence of therapeutic effects. *The International Journal of Clinical and Experimental Hypnosis, 1,* 7–20.

5. Arts

Definition. *Arts* are the various expressions of a culture; their purpose is to reflect and convey emotions or information.

Discussion. The various expressive arts considered in MindBody medicine are music, plastic arts, and acting. These have been used throughout our history to give expression to our inner selves, to the beliefs of the culture, and to bring joy and enhance social support. We offer a definition of each and a short discussion.

Music is the placing of sounds together in a melodious fashion. Music is a medium with a long history of association with healing. Both Aristotle and Pythagoras encouraged the employment of music for health, and we even have accounts of the use of music to control blood pressure during the Renaissance (Munro & Mount, 1978). Currently, music is employed in hospitals and treatment settings to help lower or eliminate stress and create states of comfort for medical procedures.

Art therapy is the expression of self through a sensible medium. Art therapy, especially painting, has been employed for many years in psychiatric hospitals as a diagnostic as well as a treatment tool (Prinshorn, 1922). It is considered a powerful tool to assist in reconciling emotional conflicts, foster self-awareness, and express unspoken and often unconscious concerns about illness

Acting is the interpreting through voice or body language a script or event. A common employment of acting in MindBody medicine has been formalized in what is called drama therapy. Drama therapy is the systematic and intentional use of drama/theater processes to achieve the therapeutic goals of symptom relief, emotional and physical integration, and personal growth

Some Areas of Application

Anxiety

Reduces and controls anxiety (Altenmueller, 2005; Guzzetta, 1989; Knight, 2001; Malchiodi, 2001; Sternberg, 2001; Yung et al., 2002).

Cardiovascular

Lowers blood pressure (Cadigan et al., 2001; Gaynos, 2000).

Dementia

Manages agitation (Remington, 2002).

End of Life

Eases the dying process (Schroeder-Sheker, 1995).

Immune System

Increases salivary immunoglobulin A (playing a percussion instrument and singing) (Kuhn, 2002).

Medical Procedures

Prepares for surgery (Rodgers, 1995; Wang, 2002; ; Sierpina, and Tuden-Neugebauer, 2004).

Use of less anesthesia and analgesic (Gaynor, 2000).

PAIN MANAGEMENT

Reduces pain (Chlan, 2001; Gaynos, 2000; Good et al., 2002).

STRESS

Lowers and controls stress in cancer patients (Cohen & Walco, 1999).

Illustrations

At our hospital (Tallahassee Memorial Health Care), children are helped to achieve the Relaxation Response (RR) through music they like. The music is played by a professional music therapist. The relaxation achieved helps the child undergo uncomfortable procedures with more comfort. In addition, increased relaxation could increase the child's T-cell activities.

Client B was 7 years old when she was in an automobile accident that killed her mother and left Client B with cuts that required two surgeries. The client became withdrawn and frightened in unfamiliar situations. Art therapy was employed to assist Client B to express her feelings, reconnect with supportive others, and be able to rework her traumatic events symbolically in a benign environment. Art therapy provided this young person with a unique means to come to terms with and accept her loss and begin to regain her self-esteem and sense of security.

SUGGESTED READING

Altenmueller, E.O. (2005). Music in your head. *Scientific American Mind,* Special Edition, 24–31. [This is an important update and review from this prestigious publication.]

Cadigan, M.E., Caruao, N.A., Halderman, S.M., et al. (2001). The effects of music on cardiac patients on bed rest. *Progress in Cardiovascular Nursing, 16,* 5–13.

Cohen, S.O., & Walco, G.A. (1999). Dance/movement therapy for children and adolescents with cancer. *Cancer Practice, 7,* 34–42. [This article is a good introduction for those not familiar with the area of applying dance to physical health. This might help you think in terms of what it is about dance therapy that is MindBody and what is simply physical.]

Gaynor, M. (2000). *The Sounds of Healing.* Random House, New York.

Good, M., Anderson, G. C., Stanton-Hicks, M., et al. (2002). Relaxation and music reduce pain after gynecologic surgery. *Pain Management Nursing, 3,* 61–70.

Guzzetta, C. (1989). Effects of relaxation and music therapy on patients in a coronary care unit with presumptive acute myocardial infarction. *Heart Lung, 18,* 609–616.

Knight, W.E. (2002). Relaxing music prevents stress-induced increases in subjective anxiety, systolic blood pressure, and heart rate in healthy males and females. *Journal of Music Therapy, 38,* 254–272. [This article will assist you in obtaining a basic grasp of the field of music therapy.]

Kuhn, D. (2002). The effects of active and passive participation in musical activity on the immune system as measured by salivary immunoglobulin. *Journal of Music Therapy, 39*, 30–39.
Malchiodi, C. (2001). Art therapy. In N. Allison (Ed.), *The Complete Body, Mind, and Spirit* (pp. 311–312). New York: McGraw-Hill.
Munro, S., & Mount, B. (1978). Music therapy in palliative care. *Cancer Medicine Association Journal, 119*, 1029–1034.
Prinshorn. (1992). *Artistry of the Mentally Ill* in *Alternative Medicine: Expanding Medical Horizons.* (National Institutes of Health report). Washington, DC: U.S. Government Printing Office.
Remington, R. (2002). Calming music and hand massage with agitated elderly. *Nursing Research, 51*, 317–323.
Rodgers, L. (1995). Music for surgery. *Advances, 11*, 49–56.
Schroeder-Sheker. (2006). *The Luminous Wound.* In press
Sierpina, V.. & Tuden-Neugebauer, C. (2004). Selected research on music in the preoperative period. Online at: cam.utmb.edu/resources/Curriculum/musicMind-BodyMedicine.pdf
Sternberg, P. (2001). Drama therapy. In N. Allison (Ed.), *The Complete Body, Mind, Spirit* (pp. 318–320). New York: McGraw-Hill.
Wang, S.M. (2002). Music and preoperative anxiety. A randomized controlled study. *Journal of Anesthesia and Analgesia, 94*, 1489–1494. [This is useful research for implementation in hospital and outpatient surgical clinics.]
Yung, P.M., et al. (2002). A controlled trial of music and pre-operative anxiety in Chinese men undergoing transurethral resection of the prostate. *Journal of Advanced Nursing, 39*, 352–359.

6. *Biofeedback*

Definition. *Biofeedback* is the practice of monitoring physical or mental activity with instruments to give an observer, usually the patient who is being monitored, information about physical or mental data of which they are normally not aware.

Discussion. Any mental or physical process or change that can be monitored can be used for biofeedback. This can range from a simple item sensitive to body heat that will change color when a person is under stress to sophisticated electrical equipment that records and reports subtle changes in the mental or physical activity. The following are the types of approaches that are used in biofeedback:

- Electromyographic: Measures muscle tension.
- Thermal: Measures skin temperatures as an indication of blood flow change.
- Electrodermal: Measures changes in sweat activity too small to feel.
- Finger pulse: Measures pulse rate and force.

- Breathing: Measures breath rate, volume, rhythm, and location (chest or abdomen).
- Neurofeedback: Measures brain wave activity (note that some authorities consider this a separate intervention since it is presumably measuring neural activity directly rather than body activity).
- Autogenic feedback training: Focuses attention on different areas of the body and induces a MindBody shift in those areas.

Some Areas of Application

Cardiovascular

Lowers blood pressure in hypertensive patients (Canino, Cordona, et al., 1994; Nako, Nomaron, et al., 1997; Nako, Nomura, Shimosawa, Fujita, & Kuboki, 1999).

Increases heart rate variability in patients with coronary artery disease (Del Pozo et al., 2004).

Headaches

Treats and sometimes eliminates headaches (Goleman, 1995; Sarafine, 2000; Schwartz & Andrasik, 2006).

Intestinal

Improves fecal incontinence (Enck, 1992 ; Guillemont et al., 1994).

Improves constipation (Heymen et al., 1999; Rao & Enck, 1997).

Skin

Reduces the severity and recurrence of psoriasis (Goodman, 1994; Polenghi et al., 1994).

Urinary Incontinence

Increases urinary continence after radical prostatectomy (McDowell et al., 1999; Van Kampen et al., 2000).

Illustrations

To eliminate migraine headache, the therapist places temperature sensors on a patient's fingers and toes. The patient is trained to be aware of the temperature information feedback and how they can influence their headache pain by warming their fingers and toes. As the patient becomes more accurate in this effort, they learn to increase the temperature without using the instruments (Schwartz & Schwartz, 1993).

Patients who underwent radical prostatectomy were trained using biofeedback to control urinary urgency and compared to a control group who did not receive biofeedback training. After 1 year, 14% more of the treatment group were still able to control their urinary urgency (Van Kampen et al., 2000).

A client of the second author is practicing autogenic feedback training. The client is seated comfortably in a chair. The client is focusing first on the lower, then upper extremities and telling himself five to seven times: "My legs are very heavy." Then, the client repeats seven times: "My arms are very heavy." The client will feel very relaxed and can continue to include other parts of the body. As the client feels this relaxation taking place, he is experiencing feedback from his body that he is accomplishing by relaxation. It is recommended to do this exercise for about 20 minutes and to close the exercise by placing a hand on the forehead and repeating five to seven times: "My forehead feels very cool." The client should experience a feeling of "coolness and freshness" as a part of feeling very relaxed.

SUGGESTED READING

Canino, E., Cordona, R., et al. (1994). A behavioral treatment program as a therapy in the control of primary hypertension. *Acta Cientific Venezolana, 45,* 23–30.

Del Pozo, J.M., et al. (2004). Biofeedback treatment increases heart rate variability in patients with known coronary artery disease. *American Heart Journal, 147,* E11. [This study sets the groundwork for demonstrating that biofeedback has the potential to be utilized for improving cardiac morbidity and mortality rates.]

Enck, P. (1992). Biofeedback training in disordered defecation. *Digestive Disease, 38,* 1953–1960.

Goleman, D., & Gurin, J. (1993). *Mind Body Medicine.* Yonkers, NY: Consumer Reports Books. [This is an excellent all-around anthology to introduce someone to MindBody medicine. In fact, this work inspired Dr. Rotan to develop his graduate seminar on the topic.]

Goodman, M. (1994). An hypothesis explaining the successful treatment of psoriasis. *Thermal Biofeedback and Self-Regulation, 19,* 347–352.

Guillemont, F., et al. (1994). Biofeedback for the treatment of fecal incontinence. *Diseases of the Colon and Rectum, 38,* 393–397. [This is a good report on the power of biofeedback when compared to medicine.]

Heymen, S., Wexner, S.D., Vickers, D., Nogueras, J.J., Weiss, E.G., & Pikarsky, A.L. (1999). Prospective randomized trial comparing four biofeedback techniques for patients with constipation. *Disease of the Colon and Rectum, 42,* 1388–1393.

McDowell, B.J., et al. (1999). Effectiveness of behavioral therapy to treat incontinence in homebound older adults. *Journal of the American Geriatrics Society, 47,* 309–318. [This is an important reference for clinicians working with the geriatric population.]

Nako, M., Nomaron, S., et al. (1997). Clinical effects of blood pressure biofeedback treatment on hypertension by auto shaping. *Psychosomatic Medicine, 59,* 331–338. [This is an important reference for clinicians working in medical settings.]

Nako, M., Nomura, S., Shimosawa, T., Fujita, T., & Kuboki, T. (1999). Blood pressure treatment, organ damage and sympathetic activity in mild hypertension. *Psychotherapy and Psychosomatics, 68,* 341–347. [Both reports by Nako et al. are significant in helping establish biofeedback as a reliable source of Mind-Body interventions instead of constant reliance on medicine.]

Polenghi, M.M., et al. (1994). Experience with psoriasis in a psychosomatic dermatology clinic. *Acta Dermato Venereologica Supplementum* (Stockholm), *186,* 65.

Rao, S., & Enck, P. (1997). Biofeedback therapy for defecation disorders. *Digestive Disorder, 15,* 78–92.

Sarafine, E. (2000). Age comparison in acquiring biofeedback control and success in reducing headache pain. *Annals of Behavior Medicine, 2,* 10.

Schwartz, M., & Andrasik, F. (2006). *Biofeedback: A Practitioner's Guide.* New York: Gulford. [This book provides an excellent overview of biofeedback.]

Schwartz, M., & Schwartz, N. (1993). Biofeedback using the body signals. In Goleman, D., & Gurin, J. (Eds.), *Mind Body Medicine.* Yonkers, New York: Consumers Report Books. 301–314.

Van Kampen, M., et al. (2000). Effect of pelvic-floor re-education on duration and degree of incontinence after radical prostatectomy: A randomized controlled trial. *Lancet, 355,* 98–102..

7. Yoga

Definition. *Yoga* is the joining of body, mind, and spirit through breathing, movement, or focus.

Discussion. In Hindu spiritual texts, yoga means a union. It refers to the joining of the individual human spirit with the motivating spirit of the universe. Note that traditionally there are nine systems of yoga: raja, hatha, mantra, yantra, kundalini, jhana, bhakti, karma, and tantric. There are three modern yoga developments: integral, Iyengar, and Kripalu. Most of the research on yoga is on the employment of hatha yoga for healing. Hatha is the path of bodily mastery and includes *asanas* (postures), *kriyas* (cleansing the integral body), and *pranayama* (breath).

Some Areas of Application

Asthma

Lowers the number of asthma attacks (Nagarathna & Nagendra, 1985).

Pain Management

Iyengar relieves stress and physical pain (Garfinkel et al., 1999).

Reduces back pain and improves back functioning (Sherman, Cherkin, Erro, et al., 2005; Williams, Petroni, Smith, et al., 2005).

IMPROVES RANGE OF MOTION

Increases range of motion in carpal tunnel syndrome (Garfinkel et al., 1999).

RESPIRATION

Minimizes asthmatic symptoms and reduces number of attacks (Vedanthar et al., 1998).

Illustrations

A patient with high blood pressure keeps her blood pressure normalized with daily practice (1 hour) of hatha yoga. Patients with carpal tunnel syndrome improve their grip after special training in Hatha Yoga (Garfinkel, 1999).

After 12 weeks of training in yoga, 101 subjects experienced less back pain and had increased their comfort and expanse of motion without medication. This was significantly different from a control group using exercise. (Sherman et al., 2005).

SUGGESTED READING

Garfinkel, M., et al. (1999). Yoga based intervention for carpal tunnel syndrome. *Journal of the American Medical Association, 280,* 1601–1603.

Nagarathna, R., & Nagendra, H.R. (1985). Yoga for bronchial asthma: A controlled study. *British Medical Journal Clinical Research ED, 291,* 1077–1079. [Although the age of this study would preclude it from this book, we felt the research design and health topic significant for inclusion. This is a rawer randomized controlled clinical trial in this area.]

Sherman, K.J., Cherkin, D.C., Erro, J., et al. (2005). Comparing yoga, exercise, and a self-care book for chronic low back pain: a randomized, controlled trial. *Annals of Internal Medicine, 143,* 849–856. [A well-done report on what seems to be careful research and cautious conclusions.]

Vedanthar, P.K., et al. (1998). Clinical study of yoga techniques in university students with asthma: A controlled study. *Allergy/Asthma Procedures, 19,* 3–9, 29.

Williams, K., Petroni, J., Smith, D., et al. (2005). Effect of Iyengar yoga therapy for chronic low back pain. *Pain, 115,* 107–117.

8. Positive Self-Talk

Definition. *Positive self-talk* involves the positive words, sentences, and inner dialogue we use to label and interpret our thoughts, feelings, beliefs, and experiences.

Discussion. The intervention of positive self-talk can be practiced by everyone. A positive inner dialogue can be very helpful and soothing for the person. The type of thoughts a person has and what the person tells him- or herself are important. A person who uses positive thoughts and focuses on positive feelings and experiences is often able to influence his or her emotional and physical well-being.

Some Areas of Application

ANXIETY

Minimizes panic attacks (Barlow, 1996).

PAIN MANAGEMENT

Eliminates the sensation of pain (Barlow, 1996; Chen, 2000).

HEALTH ENHANCEMENT

Improves sense of well-being (Holiday, 2002).

MENOPAUSE

Reduces frequency of hot flashes (Hunter & Liao, 1995).

SCHOOL PHOBIA

A regular morning routine and positive self-talk to sooth anxiety may help children to manage their school phobia (Ashford, LeCroy, & Lortie, 2006).

Illustrations

A young patient is taught to say "Stop" when anxious thoughts occur, and replaces them with a set of positive statements. This simple exercise replaces catastrophic thinking and reduces anxiety (Chen, 2000).

A patient with pain is taught to tell herself that the sensations of discomfort are the warm heat of the sun and her body's attempts to make her well. This minimizes the sensation as pain and reframes it into something positive.

A student in MindBody medicine tells himself to "let go" of any negative thought that may come up when talking about a traumatic experience with a friend.

The same student, when experiencing anxiety prior to an exam, is also taught to tell himself: "It can be done successfully; I will do my very best."

SUGGESTED READING

Ashford, J.B., LeCroy, C.W., & Lortie, K.L. (2006). *Human Behavior in the Social Environment*. Belmont, CA: Thomson Brooks/Cole.
Barlow, D.H. (1996). Advances in the psychosocial treatment of anxiety disorder. *Archives of General Psychiatry, 53*, 727–735. [Dr. Barlow is one of the top researchers and authorities on the treatment of anxiety.]
Chen, E.J.M. (2000). Behavioral and cognitive interventions in the treatment of pain in children. *Pediatric Clinics of North America, 47*, 513–525.
Holiday, S. (2002). Have fun while you can, you are only as old as you feel, don't even get old. An examination of memorable messages about aging. *Journal of Communication, 52*, 681–697.
Hunter, M.S., & Liao, K.L.M. (March 1995). *Evaluation of a four session cognitive behavioral intervention for menopausal hot flashes.* Paper presented at the British Psychological Society annual conference.

9. Energy Focus

Definition. *Energy focus* is the conscious and explicit focus of energy toward healing or preventing a problem. The energy utilized can be that of the patient, the healer, or other (e.g., God, cosmos, an object, etc.). This approach may be as informal as the healer or client consciously focusing healing energy toward a patient (e.g., the healer envisions a healing color shrinking a patient's tumor), or the approach may be formalized. The following is a list of the more formalized approaches: healing science, healing touch, huna, mari-el, natural healing, qigong, SHEN therapy, therapeutic touch. (Note that some authors include prayer in this category; we treat prayer separately.)

Discussion. A person who consciously and explicitly focuses on a specific area of his or her body that needs to be healed may be able to influence the self-healing power (e.g., increase T cells). Energy-focused healing is applied through different approaches. Therapeutic touch is practiced in holistic nursing care.

Some Areas of Application

Anxiety

Eliminates and controls phobias (Gallo, 1998).
Controls and manages performance anxiety (Gallo, 1999).
Lowers anxiety in hospitalized patients (Spielberger, Gorsuch, et al., 1998).

Pain

Decreases and eliminates the perception of pain (Keller, 1993).

Stress Reduction

Exercise (behavior) improves mental clarity and emotional stability (mind) as well as energy level and cardiovascular capacity (body) (Schafer, 1996).

Wounds

Increases rate of healing and lowers pain perception (L. Dossey, 1999; Wirth, 1990).

Illustrations

A therapeutic touch practitioner focused energy via her hands a few inches away from surgical wounds with the intention to heal them. In a controlled, double-blind study, 57% of the subjects were completely healed on Day 16, and none of the control subjects were healed (Wirth, 1990).

A 5-year-old girl who suffers asthma attacks received a 15-minute therapeutic touch session and felt free of respiratory distress. The girl expressed to the nurse who performed the session that she felt well and happy again (B. M. Dossey, Keega, & Guzzetta, 2000).

SUGGESTED READING

Dossey, L. (1999). *Reinventing Medicine: Beyond Mind Body to a New Area of Healing.* San Francisco: Harper.

Gallo, F. (1998). *Energy Psychology.* Boca Raton, FL: CRC Press. [This book is an excellent resource for any practitioner, student, or teacher.]

Keller, E. (1993). *The effects of therapeutic touch on tension headache pain.* Master's thesis, University of Missouri, Columbia.

Schafer, W. (1996). *Stress Management for Wellness.* Orlando, FL: Holt, Rinehart & Winston.

Spielberger, C.D., Gorsuch, R.L., et al. (1998). *Manual for the State-Trait Anxiety Inventory.* Palo Alto, CA: Consulting Psychologists Press.

Wirth, D. (1990). The effect of non-contact therapeutic touch on the healing rate of full-thickness surgical wounds. *Subtle Energies, 1,* 1–20.

10. Support Groups

Definition. *Support groups* involve professionally led psychotherapeutic interactions of three to nine people to assist them in managing health situations.

Discussion. The gathering of group members for the purpose of sharing, exchanging, and supporting each other in managing similar health concerns or situations can be therapeutic. The gathering is usually done within a specific time frame and on a regular basis. Support groups are economical and therefore are often encouraged by health maintenance organization providers.

Some Areas of Application

Arthritis

Decreases pain and provides a reduced treatment cost of $148 per person (Mazonson et al., 1993).

Asthma

Reduces acute asthma visits to physician for medical treatment 49% (Wilson et al., 1993).

Cancer

Extends life expectancy in breast cancer (Cain et al., 1986; Classen et al., 2001; Cunningham & Tocco, 1989; Dittmann, 2003; Fawzy, 1995; Richardson et al., 1990; Spiegel, 1998).

Extention of life expectancy in melanoma (Fawzy, 1993).

Depression

Decreases loneliness related to depression (*National Psychologist*, 2003).

Psychosomatic Problems

Eliminates complaints or lowers frequency of complaints (Hellman et al., 1990).

Illustrations

When children or adults with asthma meet in small groups on a regular basis such as one time per month, physician visits about their asthma problems and days of school absence, is reduced (Wilson et al., 1993).

Psychological self-help techniques or strategies are important for survival in patients with metastatic cancer. Patients meeting in weekly group psychological therapy over a period of 1 year and using psychological self-regulation strategies such as relaxation, mental images, cognitive restructuring, and meditation are more likely to survive metastatic cancer according to one study (Cunningham, Phillips, Lockwood, Hedley, & Edmonds, 2000).

Bereavement support groups for children and adults are very important for healing and are often set up at local hospice settings.

Support groups for persons who want to stop smoking are encouraged by community leaders and health maintenance organizations.

SUGGESTED READING

Cain, E.N., et al. (1986). Psychosocial benefits of a cancer support group. *Cancer, 57,* 183–189.

Classen, C., et al. (2001). Supportive-expressive group therapy and distress in patients with metastatic breast cancer. A randomized clinical intervention trial. *Archive of General Psychiatry, 58,* 494–501. [This article provides excellent evidence-based information.]

Cunningham, A.J., Phillips, C., Lockwood, G.A., Hedley, D.W., & Edmonds, C.V.I. (2000). Association of involvement in psychological self-regulation with longer survival in patients with metastatic cancer: An exploratory study. *Advances in Mind-Body Medicine, 16,* 176–294. [This is an excellent exploratory study that should be replicated in many health care settings with an oncology department.]

Cunningham, A.J., & Tocco, E.K. (1989). A randomized trial of group psychoeducational therapy for cancer patients. *Patient Education and Counseling, 14,* 101–114.

Dittmann, M. (2003). Coping with cancer through social connection. *Monitor on Psychology, 12,* 24–26. [This author points out the impact social connections might have on coping and recovery from cancer.]

Fawzy, F.I. (1995). Critical review of psychosocial intervention and cancer care. *Archives of General Psychiatry, 52,* 100–1300.

Fawzy, F. (1993). Malignant melanoma. *Archives of General Psychiatry, 50,* 681–689.

Hellman, C.J., et al. (1990). The study of the effectiveness of two group behavioral medicine interventions for patients with psychosomatic complaints. *Behavioral Medicine, 16,* 165–175.

Mazonson, L., et al. (1993). Evidence suggesting that health education for self management in patients with chronic arthritis has sustained health benefits while reducing health care cost. *Arthritis and Rheumatism, 36,* 439–446.

Richardson, J.L., et al. (1990). Support group. *Journal of Clinical Oncology, 8,* 356–364.

Spiegel, D. (1998). Support group. *Public Health Reports, 110,* 298.

Wilson. S.R., & Scamages, P. (1993). A controlled trial of two forms of self-management education for adults with asthma. *American Journal of Medicine. 94,* 564–576

11. Humor and Laughter

Definition. *Humor* is the quality of being laughable or comical. *Laughter* is the ability to express emotion, typically mirth, by a series of inarticulate sounds, characterized by the mouth open in a smile.

Discussion. Laughter can be practiced by everyone. There is no limit on time or when or how to laugh. Laughter is universal; it has no cultural barrier, and it is practiced by all ethnic groups. Laughter might also be used by some people as a way of coping with difficult situations.

Some Areas of Application

Cancer

Humor influences positive effects on patients with cancer (Christie & Moore, 2005).

Insomnia

Norman Cousins, author of *Anatomy of an Illness*, discovered that for every 10 minutes of hearty laughter he could sleep pain free for 2 hours (Cousins, 1981).

Immune Disorders

Increases natural killer cells and decreases stress hormones (Bennett, 2006; Beck, 1996; Fry, 1992).

Health

Humor and laughter may influence health (Bennett & Lengacher, 2006).

Stress

Reduces stress levels (Bennett, Zeller, Rosenberg, & McCann, 2003; Martin, 2003).

Palliative Care

Laughter makes good medicine for very sick patients (Sobel, 2006).

Humor is used in palliative care (Dean & Gregory, 2005).

Humor has an impact on patients with cancer (Christie & Moore, 2005).

Illustrations

Researchers at the University of California in Irvine found that expecting a happy, funny event can raise levels of endorphins and other pleasure- and relaxation-inducing hormones and lower production of stress hormones.

Researchers at the University of Maryland report that people who used humor were less likely to have heart attacks (Beck & Tan, 1996).

Humor and laughter can be therapeutic, and this belief has received varying levels of support from the scientific community at different points in its history. Current research indicates that using humor is well accepted by the public and is frequently used as a coping mechanism (Bennett & Lengacher, 2006).

Terminal illness is often accompanied by circumstances of anxiety, fear, and sadness. Hospice/palliative care emphasizes quality of life and the importance of human relationships. Hospice patients, family members, and caregivers use humor and laughter to cope with stressful events (Dean & Gregory, 2005). For example, family members bring a friend who tells humoristic jokes. Caregivers bring humorous movies for their loved ones to view.

Improvements in pain thresholds and elevations in natural killer cell activity consistently appear in quantitative experimental studies. In addition, measurements of specific neuroendocrine and stress hormone levels reveal biochemical changes that suggest improved physical stress responses and increased feelings of well-being after humorous interventions (Christie & Moore, 2005).

SUGGESTED READING

Beck, A.T., & Tan, S. (1996). Report on psychoneuroimmunology. *Research Society Meeting.*

Bennett, M.P., & Lengacher, C. A. (2006). Humor and laughter may influence health. I. History and background. *Evidence-Based Complementary and Alternative Medicine, 3*, 61–63.

Bennet, M.P., Zeller, J. M., Rosenberg, L., & McCann, J. (2003). Alternative therapies in health and medicine. *Advances , 9*, 38–45.

Cousins, N. (1981). *Anatomy of an Illness*, Bantam Books, New York. [A classic on humor and health.]

Dean, R.A., & Gregory, D.M. (2005). More than trivial: Strategies for using palliative care. *Cancer Nursing, 28*, 292–300. [This work highlights the importance of palliative interventions as well as curative ones.]

Fry, W. (1992). The physiological effects of humor mirth and laughter. *Journal of the American Medical Association*, 267, 1857–1858.

Sobel, R.K. (2006). Does laughter make good medicine? *New England Journal of Medicine*, 354, 1114–1115. [This article is an excellent resource for obtaining a deeper understanding of the entire area of humor and laughter in healing.]

12. Expressive Writing

Definition. *Expressive writing* is the venting of emotions and cognitions through words and stories.

Discussion. Writing is a form of personal expression of the "self." For instance, for a woman who is living with the reality of breast cancer, expressive writing could be a way of expressing certain feelings from her dreams or daily experiences. Expressive writing could give this person a symbolic way of exploring her personal and cultural viewpoints. Her cancer could also be understood as both an opportunity and a demand for individuation and for coping with her life-threatening situation (Greer, 2001). Impressive writing is not just keeping a record of data. It includes the writers' themselves telling about the topic.

Some Areas of Application

Arthritis

Improves range of motion (Smyth et al., 1999).

Asthma

Reduces symptoms in patients with asthma or rheumatoid arthritis (La Puma, 1999).

Breast Cancer

Explores symbolic significance of cancer (Greer, 2001).

Depression

Decreases depression (Lepore, 1997).

Stress

Relieves stress (Eng, Fitzmaurice, et al., 2003; Ulrich & Lutgendorf, 2002).

Trauma

Reduces visits to physicians and pain (Pennebaker, 1997; Smyth, 1998).

Illustrations

A person with depression writes his or her thoughts and feelings about sadness and hopelessness in life in a daily journal. The daily journal writing helps the person to ventilate his or her feelings and thoughts and increases the immune function (Lepore, 1997).

A clinical mental health care worker encourages a client to stop the negative self-talk by changing any negative thought into a positive thought and writing down only the positive thoughts.

SUGGESTED READING

Eng, P. M., Fitzmaurice, G., et al. (2003). Anger expression and risk of coronary artery disease among male health professionals. *Psychosomatic Medicine, 65,* 100–110. [These authors talk about important information for reducing stress.]

Greer, P. (2001). Breast cancer: Imaginal realms of meaning. *Journal of Poetry Therapy, 14.*

La Puma, C. (June 1999). Writing therapy to reduce asthma and RA symptoms. *Alternative Medicine Alert.*

Lepore, S.J. (1997). Expressive writing moderates the relation between intrusive thoughts and depressive symptoms. *Journal of Personality and Social Psychology, 73,* 1030–1037.

Pennebaker, J.W. (1997). *Opening Up: The Healing Power of Expressing Emotions.* New York: Guilford Press.

Smyth, J.M. (1998). Written emotional expression: Effect size, outcome types, and moderating variables. *Journal of Counseling and Clinical Psychology, 66,* 174–184.

Smyth, J.M, & Stone, N.A. (1999). Effect of writing about stressful experiences on symptom reduction in patients with asthma and rheumatoid arthritis: A randomized trial. *Journal of the American Medical Association, 14,* 1304–1309.

Ulrich, P.M., & Lutgendorf, S.K. (2002). Journaling about stressful events: Effects of cognitive processing and emotional expression. *The Society of Behavioral Medicine, 24.*

13. Poetry

Definition. *Poetry* creates images through word connection.

Discussion. Poetry is usually practiced by people who are interested in it. However, somebody does not need to know how to write poetry to use poetry. People write poetry for different reasons. Poetry is also universal, meaning different cultures use poetry in different ways. Poetry can also be used in psychotherapy to help people cope with difficult life situations.

Some Areas of Application:

ASTHMA

Reduces symptoms (La Puma, 1999).

EMOTIONAL DIFFICULTIES AND ABUSE

Reduces emotional tension in patients who experience high levels of stress (Ospina-Kammerer, 1999).

BEREAVEMENT

Assists in dealing with death and loss (Mazza, 2001).

DEPRESSION

Reduces depression (Lepore, 1997).

RHEUMATOID ARTHRITIS

Reduces symptoms (La Puma, 1999).

Illustrations

Poetry is used in hospitals, hospice facilities, mental health centers, runaway shelters, homeless shelters, and schools. Writing a poem could help a person to reflect on thoughts and feelings. The person might experience empowerment through gaining control over unresolved life issues. Poetry therapy can help a person who feels overwhelmed to restore a sense of order. Poetry therapy is not only advancing art and science, but also, more importantly, is advancing the human connection while instilling hope and giving a person a positive outlook in life (Mazza, 2003).

SUGGESTED READING

La Puma, C. (1999). Writing therapy to reduce asthma and RA symptoms. *Alternative Medicine Alert.*

Lepore, S.J. (1997). Expressive writing moderates the relation between intrusive thoughts and depressive symptoms. *Journal of Personality and Social Psychology, 73,* 1030–1037.

Mazza, N. (2001). The place of the poetic in dealing with death and loss. *Journal of Poetry Therapy, 15,* 29–35.

Mazza, N. (2003). Editor's note: The foundation and future of scholarship in poetry therapy. *Journal of Poetry Therapy, 16,* 1–4. [This author is one of the top experts in the field of poetry therapy in the United States.]

Ospina-Kammerer, V. (1999). *Poetry Therapy Within a Therapist's Practice Model.* Human Sciences, Springer Netherlands Press.

14. Prayer

Definition. *Prayer* is a request, expressions of gratitude, or praise made to another. Most studies focus on prayers of request.

Discussion. Prayer is arguably the most controversial of the MindBody interventions. This seems to be because of its association with faith, religion, and belief in a power greater than ourselves (usually a deity). Indeed, many people who use prayer do have a religious faith or belief in a deity to whom they pray. However, it is important in the study of prayer that, from a scientific point of view, there need be no presumption about a deity. From a scientific view, study of prayer is the simple exploration of the hypothesis regarding whether this phenomenon described as prayer seems to influence or be associated with a particular result. Prayers should be studied as any other MindBody intervention without any presumptions. As with many MindBody interventions, there is the element of belief or faith in its power such as there often is in interventions of physical medicine.

Many questions remain in the study of prayer. Like most interventions in MindBody medicine, prayer especially is controversial. Many of the research reports have been challenged for lack of scientific rigor. There are also reports in the literature of research that show that there is no change with prayer.Like the reports supporting prayer, we have found that these reports also have flaws in their methodology.

This is an area in which we need to know more about the variables involved when we say "prayer" for there are various types of prayers and prayer processes. This is one of the many exciting areas in MindBody medicine that offers the possibility of great exploration.

Some Areas of Application

AIDS

Decreases AIDS-related illness, severity of related illness, visits to a physician, hospitalization, and days in the hospital (Sicher et al., 1998; Targ & Taylor, 2001).

Cardiac Surgery

Pre- and postoperatively supports the person's healing process (Byrd, 1988; Harris et al., 1999).

Enhances recovery by decreasing depression and distress (Ai, 1998).

Pregnancy

Seems to be associated with positive outcomes in in vitro fertilization (Cha, Wirth, & Lobo, 2001).

Mental Health

In common with healing, searches for wholeness (Slattery, 1999).

Rheumatoid Arthritis

Lessened pain and improved mobility in prayed-for group compared to control group (Mathews, 2000).

Illustrations

A group of AIDS patients are prayed for 1 hour a day, 6 days a week for 10 weeks. The prayed-for group developed fewer AIDS-related illnesses, had fewer physician visits, and had fewer hospitalizations; when they were ill, their illness was less debilitating and their hospitalization days were fewer compared to a control group who did not receive prayer (Sicher et al., 1998).

Sense prayer carries such controversy and questions, we have included two recent studies that report a finding of no influence of prayer in healing. Note that these studies refer to standardized remote prayer (Benson, 2006; Masters, 2006).

SUGGESTED READING

Ai, A.L., Dunkle, R.E., Peterson, C., & Bolling, S.F. (1998). The role of private prayer in psychological recovery among midlife and aged patients following cardiac surgery. *Gerontologist* 38, 591–601.

Byrd, R. (1988). *Southern Medical Journal, 7,* 826–828. [This is the "classical" work on prayer and the first to attempt to employ the scientific method in prayer research. Note, however, that this study included 30 dependent variables and found significant effects, without using appropriate statistical analysis for multiple correction, for only 7 of them.]

Benson, H., Dusek, J., Bethea, C., Carpenter, H., & Rollins, S. (2006). *American Heart Journal.* [This report found that a preformed standardized prayer offered at certain times each day seemed to have no effect on prevention of complications during or after surgery.]

Cha, K.Y., Wirth, D.P., & Lobo, R.A. (2001). Does prayer influence the success of in vitro fertilization-embryo transfer? Report of a masked, randomized trial. *Journal of Reproductive Medicine, 46,* 781–787.

Harris, W.S., et al. (1999). A randomized, controlled trial of the effects of remote, intercessory prayer on outcomes in patients admitted to the coronary care unit. *Archive Internal Medicine, 159,* 2273–2278. [This work presents impressive use of the scientific method in an area in which the variables are difficult to control.]

Masters, K., Spiklmans, G., & Goodson, J. (2006). Are there demonstrable effects of distant intercessory prayer? A meta-analytic review. *Annals of Behavioral Medicine* 32, 21–26. [This study did not include prayer for oneself or prayer in the presence of the one being prayed for.]

Mathews, D., et al. (2000). Effects of intercessory prayer on patients with rheumatoid arthritis. *Southern Medical Journal.* 93, 1177–1186

Sicher, F., et al. (1998). A randomized double-blind study of the effects of distant healing in a population of advanced AIDS. *Western Journal of Medicine, 169,* 356–363. [This article is provides a better understanding of valuable research methods in prayer research.]

Slattery, D.P. (1999). Poetry, prayer and meditation. *Journal of Poetry Therapy, 13,* 39–45.

Targ, E., & Taylor, S.E. (2001). Prayer and distant healing positive and negative beliefs and the course of AIDS. *Advances in Mind-Body Medicine, 17,* 44–72.

15. Relaxation Response (RR)

The RR is a psychophysiological event manifested by parasympathetic responses (i.e., a state of relaxation). Herbert Benson (Benson, 1975, 2001; 1984) illustrates this response by a focused meditation using a word or prayer as a mantra: Meditation is the intervention; the RR is the result. Since the RR is the outcome of MindBody interventions that bring about parasympathetic response, it is a factor in all those interventions (e.g., when you employ imagery, hypnosis, meditation, etc. to bring about a parasympathetic state, you are employing the RR). Since the RR is part of so many MindBody interventions, we do not include it as a special section (Goleman, 1953).

SUGGESTED READING

Benson, H., Beary, J.F., & Carol, M.P. (1974). The relaxation response. *Psychiatry, 37,* 37–46.

Benson, H. (1975, 2001). *The Relaxation Response.* New York: Morrow.

Benson, H. (1984). *Beyond the Relaxation Response.* New York: Times Books.

Goleman, D., & Gurin J. (Eds.). (1993). *Mind Body Medicine: How to Use Your Mind for Better Health.* (pp. 233–258). Yonkers, NY: Consumer Reports Books.

Kanji, N. (2004). Autogenic training reduces anxiety after coronary angioplasty: A randomized clinical trial. *American Heart Journal, 147,* E10. [An excellent example of the RR.]

D. EXERCISE

Match the intervention to the possible results of that intervention; note to help in your learning, we have listed the definition of some interventions rather than the name of the intervention. This makes you employ more mental activity in double checking yourself. *More than one answer is possible in many cases.*

Carefully review this chapter, especially Section C, where you will find the answers to these exercise questions. It will also serve you well to commit to memory those interventions that are of interest to you.

Intervention

Yoga

____

____

Mental representation of a sensation

____

____

Prayer

____

____

Poetry

____

____

Humor and laughter

Psychotherapy

Positive self-talk

Biofeedback

Painting of a picture

Writing your thoughts and feelings about an experience

Support groups

Hypnosis

Meditation

Results of Interventions

Reduces anxiety
Shrinks tumors
Increases lymphocyte count and enhances natural killer cell function
Regulates and slows heart rhythm
Symptom reduction in patients with asthma or rheumatoid arthritis
Eliminates the sensation of pain
Improves range of motion
Reduces severity and recurrence of psoriasis
Seems to extend longevity and improve quality of life in patients fighting cancer
Reduces high blood pressure
Better than medication for long-term management of panic attacks
Improves irritable bowel syndrome
Increases wound healing rate
Reduces stress levels
Reduces visits to physicians and lowers perception of pain
Decreases AIDS-related illness

2

Mental Activities: A Way of Understanding MindBody Medicine

We hope the overview of MindBody interventions in Chapter 1 has strengthened your interest in the field of MindBody medicine. These powerful interventions focus on employing the mind to become a positive influence on our health. In Chapter 2, we consider just how this influence on our health might happen and propose a way of understanding what the mind does that brings about this influence. We propose that the mental activities such as perception, belief, memory, willing, and the like are the media by which the mind influences health and well-being. By specifying mental activities by name, we intend to improve the accuracy of MindBody interventions. For example, to talk about changing a person's belief (a mental activity) by MindBody interventions seems to us more accurate than talking about changing their thinking. Observe that *belief* is a more specific activity than just the general term *thinking*. Our intention is that this level of specificity will improve the accuracy of MindBody interventions as well as deepen the potential of MindBody research. This seems a more useful approach than attempting to work with more abstract terms like *thinking*. This chapter helps clarify this concept of "mental activity" (the term *"mental activity"* was coined by the first author).

A. GOALS

1. To better understand mental activities.
2. To create examples of how these mental activities are part of MindBody medicine.

B. LEARNING OBJECTIVES

After working through this chapter, you will be able to:

1. List examples of mental activities you believe to be accurate.
2. Identify mental activities when working with a patient.

C. INFORMATION GUIDE

To understand and utilize the thoughts presented in Chapter 2, it is important to consider just what this thing we call *mind* does that influences our emotions and behaviors. We call what the mind does *mental activities*. Our definition of *mind* includes the concept of the ability to perform mental activities. Most of the definitions in Appendix A reflect this idea of some activity (e.g., believing, willing, thinking, remembering). In considering the variety of definitions and in attempting to make MindBody medicine more refined and scientific, we posed this question: Just what are these activities of the mind? Reason indicated that more specific ideas should be developed about these activities and how they could be employed for promoting health.

For example, if we understand that a mental activity is *belief*, could we not focus on this understanding to strengthen or change beliefs as needed to acquire or maintain health? We could better target an intervention. That means that instead of just using, for example, imagery to prepare a patient for surgery, we would be aware of and use the patient's belief system about surgery, health, recovery, and so on to target that system specifically and consciously through the use of imagery.

To clarify further, we are suggesting that by understanding the mental activities of a patient we can address those activities by applying an appropriate intervention from Chapter 1. Thus, for example, we do not just apply an intervention such as hypnosis with a focus of helping a patient stop panic attacks or control asthma. We also might employ psychotherapy or positive self-talk to address any mental activities involved in the patient's panic or asthma. Therefore, if we discover that this patient has a strong perception and belief (both mental activities) that he or she will have panic in a particular situation or that whenever there is violence in the home he or she will have an asthma attack, we address these mental activities of perception and belief to change them as part of the entire treatment. It will become more evident as you work with patients that if you do not first change some mental activities, then your MindBody interventions will not be as effective.

By better understanding these mental activities, you are able to appreciate their relationship to health and how you might employ them more accurately to affect health care. (If you understand what a car does, then you can better use it to get safely where you need to go.) In this chapter, we share some thoughts on just what are these mental activities. As you read and study the particular mental activities presented, think how a particular mental activity could be part of health and illness and how in influencing that activity you might enhance health.

This chapter presents a list of what we propose are mental activities. Following this list are illustrations of how these mental activities relate to our physical selves in normal situations as well as in situations relating specifically to health.

Mental Activities

We hypothesize that the mind:

- Perceives: the ability to be aware of the reality around us.
- Believes: the process of having conviction about something.
- Remembers: the ability to bring into awareness information previously experienced/learned.
- Imagines: the ability to create sensual representations.
- Wills: the ability to decide on an approach and desire its outcome.
- Understands: the ability to appreciate the relationships of the variables considered. This activity seems to include the ability to organize and calculate.
- Creates: the ability to develop new ways to achieve an end. Like understanding, this activity may include organizing and calculating.

Okay, so what? Remember part of our definition: MindBody medicine is the study of how mental activities … influence health. (This would be analogous to the study in physical medicine of how biochemical activities influence health.) To begin to understand how mental activities might influence our health, it is necessary to become familiar with examples of some mental activities that influence our behavior and our physical body and the type of physical reactions those activities might generate. We present simple examples of mental activities influencing the physical body and behavior (Illustration 1). Then, the focus is on enhancing your understanding of mental activities in situations relating more specifically to our health (Illustration 2). A deeper understanding of how mental activities might influence our health will then be enriched as you study Chapters 3 through 6.

Illustration 1

Illustration 1 provides examples of mental activities and how they influence behavior and our physical body (the mental activities are underlined).

> You are on a picnic. It is a beautiful day, and you and your companion are about to spread out a picnic lunch. You hear a distant noise. What's this? You perceive in the distance an animal that, as you scan your memory, sounds very much like a bull. As it comes toward you, you and your friend begin to believe that it is a bull. You might imagine all kinds of problems if you encounter a bull. You sweat, your heart beats fast, and you may even notice a slight pain in your chest. Your friend's asthma begins to assert itself. You both suddenly see much more clearly. You are organizing your thoughts and creating possibilities. Finally, you decide (an aspect of willing) to climb over a fence and out of the way. Here he comes—your bull. But, what's this? It's not a bull at all. You remember and perceive the difference and understand: This is a cow. You organize the data in your memory and believe this animal to be safe, perhaps even friendly. However, you calculate the odds of it being friendly and decide to creatively choose a new place to picnic. Although it may be slightly difficult for either of you to speak coherently for a few minutes after this incident, you notice how your heart has slowed, pain is gone, and asthma has eased.

The story illustrates mental activities that seem to affect our physical self. You and your friend were in no real danger from a bull; however, through a number of mental activities indicated in the story, your body reacted as if you were in true danger. Such recognition of mental activities and how they relate to our bodily processes (as in the story) gives us a basis for appreciating MindBody medicine.

In MindBody medicine, we study how mental activities relate to our physical activity. We are interested to know how something we think (e.g., our memory about a bull) relates to a physical response (e.g., heart beating faster, pupils dilating), which you will see are part of a sympathetic nervous response. As we establish insight into this relationship, we can form techniques to intervene for health or to prevent illness (e.g., memory of something to bring about relaxation, i.e., a parasympathetic response). The bull/cow story illustrates interactions of mental processes on the body. Having seen that these interactions occur, let us now apply this knowledge to MindBody medicine.

Illustration 2

In Illustration 2, mental activities are underlined; interventions are in *italics*.

> A patient suffers from migraine headaches and hypertension. When she believes she is at risk in a situation (going into a stranger's home), she will often develop a headache, and her blood pressure goes up. She believes that in this situation she may be disliked because she believes she is overweight. However, in spite of willing herself to go into the home, she has a physical reaction. In our work together, she is beginning to understand the reaction of her central nervous system in this situation

(she goes into a sympathetic response). We use *hypnosis, imagery,* and *music* to help her avoid the sympathetic response. She creates her own *imagery* and uses *music* she remembers to be soothing. She also believes that her work with me will help her. After she organizes her memory and perceptions and creates her *imagery,* we employ the *hypnosis, imagery,* and *music.* (These have been calculated from the data that for her, at this time, this is the best approach.) After two sessions in which she understands, perceives, and remembers what we have discussed, she is able to go into the home without the sympathetic reaction.

Review this illustration with the underlined mental functions to understand what the mind does, and that by influencing what it does we can change perception and belief about physical reality and our body's response to that reality (e.g., her image, perception, and belief about the situation is changed) through MindBody interventions *(hypnosis, imagery, music).* In the Exercise section, you are given an opportunity to identify what mental activities might influence certain behaviors.

SUGGESTED READING

Cousins, N. (1990). *Head First: The Biology of Hope and the Healing Power of the Human Spirit.* New York: Viking Penguin. [Although this is not a rigorous scientific work, Cousins is an important contributor to the field because of his emphasis on hope and expectation. His own experience bears witness to this.]

Hart, E. (1995). *Creative Loop: How the Brain Makes a Mind.* New York: Addison-Wesley.

Mannion, M. (1997). Wilhelm Reich, 1897–1957. *Alternative and Complementary Therapies,* 3, 194.

Sabaawi, M. (2004). The mind and the brain: Neuroplasticity and the power of mental force. *Journal of Child and Family Studies,* 13, 125–127.

D. EXERCISES

Critique

Activities of the mind. Does the listing of mental activities make sense to you? Commit to memory the activities you believe are true. Read the following stories and underline the mental activities that occur in the stories.

Story 1: Airplane Travel to Your Hometown

You are on an airplane. You hear a strange noise in the rear of the plane, near your seat. What's this? An image of a plane tire coming off crosses your mind. Or could it be something else? You scan your memory for anything you might have seen on television that reminded you of this strange noise. Yes, you remember a news report of an odd noise heard just before a plane had engine problems. You perceive that something is wrong. You sweat; your heart beats faster; you might even notice a slight pain in your chest. Your friend asks why you are so frightened. You tell your friend that you have been watching the news too often lately. Yes, the news influenced your mental picture. It took you a while until you understood there was nothing wrong with the plane; it was just normal air turbulence affecting the flight. You remember and perceive the difference and understand this is normal turbulence as in your previous flights. You organize the data in your memory and believe the noise to be air turbulence. You calculate the odds of it being safe and decide to relax until the plane is in flight.

Now, check your answers below, focusing on the underlined words.

Story 1 Answers

You are on an airplane. You hear a strange noise in the rear of the plane, near your seat. What's this? An image of a plane tire coming off crosses your mind. Or could it be something else? You scan your memory for anything you might have seen on television that reminded you of this strange noise. Yes, you remember a news report of an odd noise heard just before a plane had engine problems. You perceive that something is wrong. You sweat; your heart beats faster; you might even notice a slight pain in your chest. Your friend asks why you are so frightened. You tell your friend that you have been watching the news too often lately. Yes, the news influenced your mental picture. It took you a while until you understood there was nothing wrong with the plane; it was just normal air turbulence affecting the flight. You remember and perceive the difference and understand this is normal turbulence as in your previous flights. You organize the data in your memory and believe the noise to be air turbulence. You calculate the odds of it being safe and decide to relax until the plane is in flight.

However, through a number of mental activities, which you underlined in the story, your body reacted as if you were in true danger. The recognition of mental activities and how they have a relationship with our bodily processes (as in the story) gives us a basis for appreciating MindBody medicine.

Story 2: Lower Back Pain

A patient has pain in his lower back. When he perceives being at risk in his workplace (e.g., scheduled meeting with his supervisors), he will often develop lower back pain. He believes that in this situation he may be disliked because he believes he is not a good worker , and his supervisor might dislike him for that. He remembers being ridiculed as a child by his father, who would often call him a "loser." However, in spite of willing himself to meet with the supervisor, he experiences lower back pain. Through therapy, he is perceiving, believing, and understanding how his central nervous system reacts in this situation (he goes into a sympathetic response). We use *hypnosis, imagery,* and *music* to help him avoid the sympathetic response. He creates his own *imagery* and uses *music* he remembers to be soothing. He also believes that this work will help him. After he organizes his memory and perceptions and creates his desired *imagery,* the *hypnosis, imagery,* and *music* are employed, provided this is the best approach for him. After two sessions in which he understands, perceives, and remembers what we have discussed, he is able to meet with the supervisor without the sympathetic reaction. This understood victory on his part makes him less likely to tighten his lower back muscles, which would intensify his lower back pain.

Story 2 Answers

A patient has pain in his lower back. When he perceives being at risk in his workplace (e.g., scheduled meeting with his supervisors), he will often develop lower back pain. He believes that in this situation he may be disliked because he believes he is not a good worker and his supervisors might dislike him for that. He remembers being ridiculed as a child by his father, who would often call him a "loser." However, in spite of willing himself to meet with the supervisor, he experiences lower back pain. Through therapy, he is perceiving, believing, and understanding how his central nervous system reacts in this situation (he goes into a sympathetic response). We use *hypnosis, imagery,* and *music* to help him avoid the sympathetic response. He creates his own *imagery* and uses *music* he remembers to be soothing. He also believes that this work will help him. After he organizes his memory and perceptions and creates his desired *imagery,* the *hypnosis, imagery,* and *music* are employed, provided this is the best approach for him. After two sessions in which he understands, perceives, and remembers what we have discussed, he is able to meet with the supervisor without the sympathetic reaction. This understood victory on his part makes him less likely to tighten his lower back muscles, which would intensify his lower back pain.

Review this illustration with the underlined mental functions to help you understand what the mind does and that by manipulating what it does we might change physical reality (e.g., his image, perception, and belief about the situation are changed) through MindBody interventions (hypnosis, imagery, music).

Story 3: Health Story

A person perceives symptoms of a cold. When she perceives a temperature change in her body, like feelings of hot and cold, she remembers and associates (i.e., organizes) her information and decides that she is going to be ill. She remembers her supervisor telling her to get a flu shot early in the fall season. However, in spite of perceiving and believing that a flu shot can prevent a person from getting ill, she feared the needle stick.

She needed a strategy to enable her to get the flu shot. She imagines the needle as a bee sting and the vaccine as little bee soldiers protecting her from the flu. She is now perceiving, believing, and understanding the reaction of the central nervous system in this situation. Through imaging, she is helping herself avoid the sympathetic response. She creates her own image soothing her anxiety about the needle stick.

Story 3 Answers

A person perceives symptoms of a cold. When she perceives a temperature change in her body, like feelings of hot and cold, she remembers and associates (i.e., organizes) her information and decides that she is going to be ill.. She remembers her supervisor telling her to get a flu shot early in the fall season. However, in spite of perceiving and believing that a flu shot can prevent a person from getting ill, she feared the needle stick. She needed a strategy to enable her to get the flu shot. She imagines the needle as a bee sting and the vaccine as little bee soldiers protecting her from the flu. She is now perceiving, believing, and understanding the reaction of the central nervous system in this situation. Through imaging, she is helping herself avoid the sympathetic response. She creates her own image soothing her anxiety about the needle stick.

3

The Energy System: Another Way to Understand MindBody Medicine

Whether the focus is on ancient systems of healing that consider such concepts as *Chi*, *prana*, or *ki* or on modern science, which considers concepts such as the balance of chemical energy, as in pH balance or serotonin level, healing systems have long placed value on the balancing of energy. In this chapter, we ask you to consider energy's role in MindBody medicine. Chapter 3's expanded details will help build your understanding about the use of energy in healing. As you become more familiar with this information about energy, you will be invited to consider how mental activities (e.g., perception) or MindBody interventions (e.g., meditation) may interact with energy and energy systems.

A full understanding of how energy and MindBody medicine relate will, by necessity, be a challenge because there are as yet no clear answers. So, why consider this possible relationship? The answer is simply because this relationship, although still not completely understood, is already being applied in MindBody medicine as well as other approaches to healing. As authors, we felt it important to address this topic of energy early in the text to encourage your critical thinking and help you develop a deeper understanding of some of the current activity and thought surrounding it.

The Information Guide section of this chapter helps you focus on thoughts about energy and its application in MindBody medicine. We include a lengthy discussion that gives you much up-to-date information on key concepts about energy and how they may relate to healing. Although arguably not all these approaches are MindBody medicine in the strictest sense, they are included to assist your awareness of the amount of study ongoing in this area. For those with particular interest in the field, Appendix D provides more detailed energy information.

A. GOALS

1. To better understand the concept of energy systems.
2. To begin to better understand the relationship of MindBody medicine to energy.

B. LEARNING OBJECTIVES

After working through this chapter, you will be able to

1. Define energy.
2. Identify MindBody interventions that claim to use energy in MindBody medicine.
3. Relate energy systems to aspects of health and illness.

C. INFORMATION GUIDE

Energy is understood to be the ability to do work. In effect, it is the ability to influence something to change, to go from a state of potency to activity or to change focus or direction. When we start a car, the car goes from a state of potency (e.g., potentially ready to move) to a state of activity (e.g., now actually moving). Similarly, when we steer the car, we use energy to change the car's direction. Another example would be the simple act of throwing a baseball. Whatever it takes for you to throw that ball (e.g., to make it go from a state of potency, which is a static state, to moving actively) is energy. If that baseball is hit by a batter, then energy is used to change that ball's direction. In applying this to MindBody medicine, we can say that by applying certain MindBody interventions, we can be presumed to help something in the human system go from a state of potential change to a state of activation or affect a change in direction. This means we are using some kind of energy to help the patient's system go from a static state (e.g., the immune system is not reacting to an invading organism) to an active state (e.g., the immune system begins to send healing B and T cells to attack the invading organism). Energy assists the organism in going from a state of potential health to actual health. In the same way, we might employ energy to help change the direction.

Using the example of the immune system, we could say that we might change "focus" or "direction" of the immune system. This is illustrated when we utilize hypnosis and imagery to intervene in an autoimmune problem by redirecting or refocusing immune cells away from attacking the self. Another illustration would be the utilization of hypnosis to help a patient move blood in the body, thereby assisting healing of a wound.

These illustrations relate to the possibility that many MindBody interventions employ energy to activate a system or change that system's direction, whatever the intervention. This employment of energy is done without a direct focus on the idea of energy. Thus, by utilizing hypnosis to move blood, energy is employed even though energy, as such, may not be the overt focus of the intervention. In essence, there was no overt thinking about or referral to energy when the hypnotic intervention was applied.

Other approaches in MindBody medicine overtly and deliberately employ energy in healing, such as "energy focus," sometimes imagery, many times hypnosis, and more. These approaches often overtly visualize or otherwise focus energy directly, for example, the employment of hypnosis and imagery to enable a patient to visualize and focus energy on a tumor to shrink it or the "laying on" of hands with deliberate, conscious focusing of energy to heal a wound. Both instances involve the active, deliberate use of our mental activities to focus energy toward healing.

Types of Energy

It will be helpful to appreciate some different ways in which energy can be applied in various approaches to healing. Gallo (1998) states that energy exists in various states and forms, and some can be detected and measured, while others cannot. For example, certain psychotherapy (thought field therapy) can be directed successfully at a specific energy level. Gallo further hypothesizes that the utilization of an electrical, electromagnetic, or photoelectric process at a neuron synapse could be responsible for normal as well as abnormal functioning of neurotransmitters (p. 10).

The National Center for Complementary and Alternative Medicine presents us with another way of understanding energy and defines two types of energy: veritable and putative. *Veritable energy* is easily measured and commonly accepted in healing. Some examples of this energy are sound, light, magnetism, and laser beams. All these forms of energy involve the use of specific, measurable wavelengths and frequencies in health care.

Putative energy (or energy fields), although difficult or thus far impossible to measure, is believed by many practitioners and patients to be real. The acceptance of the existence of this type of energy is reflective of the belief that humans are infused with a subtle form of energy. This energy is known by several names, depending on the system of healing, including *qi* in traditional Chinese medicine, *ki* in the Japanese Kampo system, and *doshas* in Ayurvedic medicine; others use such terms as *prana, etheric, fohat, orgone, odic force,* and *mana*. Putative energy is currently the most common focus of MindBody medicine and may indeed be found to be the matrix or conduit through which mental activities are "allowed" to influence our health.

Whatever the energy, MindBody medicine is used when we employ any conscious and explicit focus of energy toward healing or preventing a problem. Remember the energy presumed to be utilized can be that of the patient, the healer, or another (e.g., God, cosmos, an object, etc.).

One area of using energy in healing is that of energy psychology. Comprehensive energy psychology has been gaining recognition since 1998 not only by clinicians, but also by the public. Energy psychology includes the following: (1) the reality of MindBody interactions; (2) more than 30 years of research about interventions with the human biofield and chakras from the therapeutic touch literature; (3) awareness of the meridians due to the acceptance of acupuncture in health care in 1997 by the National Institutes of Health, including the Federal Drug Administration; and (4) the clinical recognition that emotional distress can be created by strongly held thought patterns created by a person (for further detailed discussion of these thoughts, refer to Appendix D).

SUGGESTED READING

Benor, D.J. (2002). Energy medicine for the internist. *Medical Clinics of North America, 8,* 105–256.

Dossey, B.M., Keegan, L., & Guzzetta, C.E. (2000). *Holistic Nursing.* Gaithersburg, MD: Aspen.

Dienstfrey, H. (1996). One view of 14 responses to five questions. *Advances* 12(3), 37.

Epstein, G. (1996). *Advances. The Journal of Mind-Body Health, 12*(3).

Figely, C.R., & Carbonell, J.L. (1995). Active ingredients project: The systematic clinical demonstration of the most efficient treatments of PTSD. In F.P. Gallo (Ed.), *Energy Psychology.* Boca Raton, FL: CRC Press. pp. 18–20. [This is Florida State University psychological research of 1995, and the entire project is an important contribution to knowledge of the treatment of trauma.]

Gallo, F.P. (1998). *Energy Psychology.* Boca Raton, FL: St. Lucie Press.
Gallo's work is basic for understanding concepts of the possible employment of energy in healing.

Hover-Kramer, D. (1999). Comprehensive energy psychology: Emerging concepts for integrative psychologists. *San Diego Psychologist, 8*(5)

National Center for Complementary and Alternative Medicine. Energy Medicine an Overview. Retrieved from: http//nccam.nih.gov/health/backgrounds/energymed.htm

D. EXERCISES

1. Write out a definition of energy that you believe is useful to your understanding of MindBody medicine.

____

____

____

____

2. Speculate on which energy concepts might apply to various Mind-Body interventions (e.g., focused energy healing might use the auras as a medium for results).

____

____

____

____

3. Sensing your own energy meridians: You may practice sensing your own energy flow meridians by focusing your attention on your feet or your hands. Keep on focusing and relax into this experience, letting yourself become aware of a sense of movement like an underground river flowing quietly. According to the Chinese tradition, this energy flow goes from foot and hand to head. By practicing this exercise, you allow yourself to become more aware of your own energy.

____

____

____

____

Visualize Your Own Healing Power

1. Relax your body by using your own breathing technique.
2. Focus on a beam of light (color of your choice).
3. Place "your colored light" on the area (body or mental activity) you want to heal.
4. Set up your own healing schedule (a few times per day and per week).
5. Keep a journal and track your healing power and your health.

4

Psychosocial Phenomena That Relate to Health

Chapter 2 explored mental activities (e.g., perception). These mental activities influence our response to the world around us (e.g., if we perceive and believe we are in danger, then we have a physical response to that perception and belief whether we are truly in danger or not). There is a body of research that has isolated some of these responses and how they relate to our health and disease. This research has focused on such variables as support, stress, emotional response, thoughts, and behaviors (for simplicity, we label these variables *psychosocial phenomena*). In Chapter 4, we list some examples of these psychosocial phenomena and their relationship to health. With this information, you will be better able to predict possible problems and perhaps prevent or change situations for health. For example, by knowing a patient is under distress and knowing that distress is associated with illness, an intervention strategy might be to help the patient change or modify the stress. This will often occur by assisting them to change their mental activity (e.g., changing their belief that there is no way out of a situation to perceiving and believing that there is a way out).

A. GOAL

The goal of this chapter is learn some of the psychosocial phenomena that relate to health and illness.

B. LEARNING OBJECTIVES

After working through this chapter, you will be able to

1. Relate psychosocial phenomena to aspects of health and illness.
2. Apply information learned to a patient situation.

C. INFORMATION GUIDE

In this section, we share some examples of psychosocial phenomena that research has associated with both health and illness. As you study this section, practice applying the information to situations you have experienced (e.g., do you know someone with cancer that has or does not have social support? How does this seem to influence the person? Have you noticed any association with high stress and a compromised immune system, such as catching a cold, etc.?). At the end of the chapter are exercises to help you review and apply this information. (Keep in mind that most studies are correlational and do not necessarily indicate cause and effect; be skeptical yet open for this is how science grows.)

1. Examples of psychosocial phenomena related to good health:
   a. The perception of social support is associated with
      - Living twice as long with cancer than people without social support (Fawzy et al., 1993; Richardson & Shelton, 1990; Spira & Carlon, 2000).
      - Increase in natural killer cells (Pinus, 1994).
      - Lower risk of myocardial infarction (Rosengreen et al., 2004; Smith et al., 2002).
      - General good health (Grzywacz, 2004).
      - Increased resistance to upper respiratory infection (Doyle, Cohen, et al., 2003; Cohen, 1997).

   b. Patients who express a fighting spirit (i.e., refuse to give up, assume an attitude of defeating their illness).
      - Surviving longer with breast cancer than those who do not express this attitude (Dean, 1998; Derogatis, 1997).
      - Feel better, survive longer, and have fewer days of debilitation with any illness (Greer, 2000; Stolbach, 2003).

   c. Perception and belief that problems can be seen as opportunities or challenges rather than overwhelming phenomena and a commitment to a cause or life in general are associated with good health (Kobasa, 1982).

   d. Optimism is associated with
      - Longevity (Levy, 2002).
      - Enhanced immune system in the elderly (Ostir, 2004).
      - Improvement in cardiac health (Ornish, 2003).
      - Strengthening of the immune system (Smith, 2002).

   e. Constructive management of anger is associated with lower blood pressure in hypertensives (Davidson et al., 2002).

   f. Forgiving perceived wrongs to oneself or others is associated with healthful blood pressure (Lawler et al., 2003).

2. Examples of psychosocial phenomena associated with illness are as follows:
   a. High stress (i.e., perception and belief that a situation is "unbearable," with little or no hope) is associated with
      - Accelerating the aging process in women by shortening the life of immune cells (Academy of Science, 2004).
      - Suppressed immune system (Brosschot et al., 1994; Shavit et al., 1985).
      - Increased bone fragility in women (Kielkolt-Glaser et al., 1995).
      - Slowing of wound healing (Kielkolt-Glaser et al., 1995; Broadbent, Petrie, Alley, & Booth, 2003).
      - The common cold (Cohen, 1997; Cohen, et al., 2003).
      - Increased risk of cardiovascular disease (Esch et al., 2002; McMahon & Lip, 2002; Sheps et al., 2002; Theorell, 2005; Vathera & Kivimaki, 2004).
      - Increase in genital herpes outbreak in women with the disease (Cohen, 1999).
      - Increased blood sugar in diabetics (Surwit, 2004).
      - Decrease in plasma triglyceride clearance (Stoney, 2002).
      - Increase in cholesterol levels (Kivimake et al., 2002).
      - Tumor growth (Glasers, 1995).
      - Lower back pain (Power et al., 2001).
      - Increase in blood pressure (Yan et al., 2003).
      - Aggravation of rheumatoid arthritis (Zutra et al., 1989).
      - Increase in incidence of irritable bowel syndrome (Drossman, 2000).
   b. Anger, anxiety, and depression are associated with hypertension (Rutledge & Hogan, 2002).
   c. Hostility is associated with cardiovascular problems (Siegman, 2000).
   d. Unmanaged anger is associated with
      - Heart attack (Chang, 2002; Williams, 2000).
      - Increase in tumor necrosis factor (Swasey, 2002).
   e. Anxiety and depression are associated with
      - Hypertension (Jonas, 1997).
      - Cancer (Watson, 1998).
      - Coronary artery disease (Glassman, 1996; Ruguiles, 2002).
   f. Depression is associated with
      - Cardiovascular problems (Barefoot, 1993; Ferkelich, 2000; Glassman & Shapiro, 1998; Gump et al., 2004; Lesperance & Frasure-Smith, 2002; Van Melle, deJonge, et al., 2004; Wassertheil-Smoller 2004).
      - Preeclampsia (Kube, 2000).
      - Lowering of immune system (Irwin, 1992).
      - Increased complication of HIV symptoms (Lyketsos et al., 1993).
      - Development of cancer (Spiegel, 2003).

g. Hopelessness is associated with
   - Cancer (Greer, 2000).
   - Cardiovascular problems (Everson et al., 1996).
h. Perception of low social support and loneliness are associated with lowering of the immune system's strength and increase in diseases (Cole, 2003; Kiecolt-Glaser, 1993; Pressman & Cohen, 2005).

In general, we have concluded from our experience and the reported experience of others that illness of all types tends to be associated with depression, intense long-term distress, cancer diagnosis in spouse, death of a spouse, low social support, and jobs that are repetitive in nature, have high demands for results, and allow few options to the workers.

Further, we should consider the following when considering the psychosocial aspects of health: A person who is perceiving, believing, and understanding how his or her central nervous system reacts in a given situation is at the same time a product of the environmental, social, and economic influences. We have to recognize that there are health-affected people with cancer, immune disorders, birth defects, and asthma, just to name a few conditions that are very much influenced by the environment in which these people live or work. Researchers also challenge the MindBody movement regarding social and environmental factors that influence human beings. Henry Dreher and other critical thinkers, such as Lerner (2000), in MindBody medicine point out that clinicians need to include the environmental and societal issues of a person. For example, in the effort to prevent and undo nicotine addiction, clinicians working with clients on this addiction and using MindBody interventions would also work on a communal and societal level by speaking out about the psychosocial grip that tobacco still has in our society (Dreher, 2001). Another example in MindBody medicine is pain management for patients with chronic illnesses. MindBody interventions (e.g., imagery, meditation, biofeedback, muscle relaxation, autogenic training, psychotherapy) are very helpful in cutting back on analgesics and increase quality of life for the person who suffers pain. MindBody intervention requires time and commitment, which also means that medical centers need to include these interventions in their budgets (Dreher, 2001).

SUGGESTED READING

Academy of Science. *Proceedings of the National Academy of Science.* Retrieved November 30, 2004, from the academy Web site.

Barefoot, J. (1993). How to use your mind for better health. In *Mind Body Medicine.* Goleman, D. & Gurin, J. (Eds.). Yonkers, New York: Consumer Reports Books. pp. 68–69.

Broadbent, E., Petrie, K.J., Alley, P.G., & Booth, R.J. (2003). Psychological stress impairs early wound repair following surgery. *Psychosomatic Medicine, 65,* 865–869.

Brosschot, J.F., et al. (1994). Influence of life stress on immunological reactivity to mild psychological stress. *Psychosomatic Medicine, 56,* 216–224.

Chang, P. (2002). Angry personality increases heart attack risks fivefold. *Archives of Internal Medicine, 162,* 901–906.

Cohen, S. (1997). Psychosocial stress and susceptibility to the common cold. *New England Journal of Medicine, 325,* 606–612.

Cohen, S., Doyle, W., Shoner, D.P., Rabin, B.S., & Gwaltney, J.M. (1997). Social ties and susceptability to the common cold. *Journal of American Medical Association,* 277: 1940–1944.

Cohen, S., Doyle, W., Turner, R.B., et al. (2003). Emotional style and susceptivity to the common cold. *Psychosomatic Medicine, 65,* 652–657.

Cohen, F., Kemeny M.E., Kearney, K.A., Zegans, L.S., Neuhaus, J.M., & Conant, M.A. (1999). Persistent stress as a predictor of genital herpes recurrence. *Arch Intern Med. 159*(20), 2430–2436.

Cole, S. (2003). AIDS Institute of the University of California.

Davidson, K., et al (2002). Constructive venting behavior predicts blood pressure in a population based sample. *Health Psychology, 19,* 55–64.

Doyle, Cohen, et al. (2003). Emotional style and susceptibility to the common cold. *Psychosomatic Medicine, 65,* 652–657. [This is an excellent review article.]

Derogatis, L.R. (1997). Psychological coping mechanisms and survival time in metastatic breast cancer. *Journal of American Medical Association, 242,* 1504–1508.

Dreher, H. (2001). A challenge to the mind-body health movement. *Advances in Mind-Body Medicine, 17,* 147–150. [This author is a great thinker in MindBody medicine.]

Drossman, D.A. (2000). AGA technical review on irritable bowel syndrome. *Gastroenterology,* 123, 2108–2131.

Esch, T., Stefano, G., Fricchione, G., & Benson, H. (2002). Stress in cardiovascular disease. *Medical Science Monitor, 8,* RA93–RA101.

Everson, S.A., et al. (1996). Hopelessness and risk of mortality and incident of myocardial infarction and cancer. *Psychosomatic Medicine, 58,* 113–121.

Fawzy, F.I., et al. (1993). Malignant melanoma: Effects of an early structured psychiatric intervention. *Archives of General Psychiatry, 50,* 681–689.

Glassman, A.H., & Shapiro, P.A. (1998). Depression and the course of coronary artery disease. *American Journal of Psychiatry, 155,* 4–11.

Greer, S. (2000). Psychological response to breast cancer. *Lancet, 49.*

Grzywacz, J.C. (2004). Toward health promotion: Physical and social behavior in complete health. *American Journal of Health Behavior, 28,* 99–111. [This is an excellent review of how the mind affects the body and vice versa.]

Gump, B., et al. (2004). Depressive symptoms and mortality in men: Results from the Multiple Risk Factor Interventions Trial. *Stroke, 36,* 98–102.

Irwin, M. (1992). Depression: Central corticotropic releasing factor activates the autonomic nervous system and reduces natural killer cell activity. In N. Schneiderman et al. (Eds.), *Stress and Disease Process.* Mahwah, NJ: Erlbaum.

Jonas BS, Franks P, Ingrans DD (1997). Are symptoms of anxiety and depression risk factors for hypertension? *Archives of Family Medicine* 6:43-9.

Kielkolt-Glaser, J.K., et al. (1995). Slowing of wound healing by psychological stress. *Lancet, 346,* 1194–1196. [This article provides helpful information for clinicians.]

Kiecolt-Glaser, J.K., & Marucha, P.T. (1995). Slowing of wound healing by psychological stress. *Lancet* 346, 1194–1196.

Kivimaki, M., Leino-Arjas, P., et al. (2002). Work stress and risk of cardiovascular mortality. Prospective cohort study of industrial employees. *British Medical Journal, 19*, 7369–7375.

Kobasa, S.C., Maddi, S.R., & Puccett, M.C. (1982). Personality and exercise as buffers in the stress-illness relationship *Journal of Behavioral Medicine, 5*, 391–404.

Lawler, et al. (2003). A change of heart: Cardiovascular correlates of forgiveness in response to interpersonal conflict. *Journal of Behavioral Medicine, 5*, 373–393. [This information is very useful for psychotherapists.]

Lerner, M. (2000). Mind-body health at 25: An assessment. *Advances in Mind-Body Medicine, 16*, 295. [The authors and Lerner are challenging researchers in MindBody medicine, with ideas such as that we should never forget the "person in the context of the environment and the eco system" and how mental activities might relate to those factors.]

Lesperance, F., & Fansure-Smith, N. (2000). Depression in patients with cardiac disease. A practical review. *Journal of Psychosomatic Research, 48*, 379–391.

Lyketsos, C., et. al (1993). Depressive symptoms as predictors of medical outcomes in HIV infection. *JAMA, 270*, 2563–2567.

McMahon, K.M., & Lip, G.Y. (2002). Psychological factors in heart failure: A review of the literature. *Archives of Internal Medicine, 162*, 51–61.

Ornish, D. (2003) Toward a joyful life. *Advances* 19, 23–25.

Ostir, G.V. (2004). Onset of frailty in older adults and the protective role of positive affect. *Psychology and Aging, 19*, 402–408.

Pinus, T. (1994). Data confirm the social context of disease. *Advances, 10*, 2.

Power, C., et al. (2001). Predictors of low back pain onset in a prospective British study. *American Journal of Public Health, 91*, 1671–1678.

Pressman, S., & Cohen, S. (May 24, 2005). Loneliness, social network size, and immune response to influenza vaccine in college freshman. *Health Psychology*, 297–306.

Rosengreen, A., et al. (2004). Coronary disease in relation to social support and social class in Swedish men: A 15-year follow-up in the study of men born in 1933. *European Heart Journal, 25*, 56–63.

Richardson, J.L., Shelton, D., et al. (1990). The effect of compliance with treatment in survival among patients with hematologic malignancy. *Journal of Clinical Oncology, 8*, 356–364.

Ruguiles, R. (200). Depression as a predictor for coronary heart disease: A review and meta-analysis. *American Journal of Preventive Medicine, 23*, 51–61.

Rutledge, T., & Hogan, B.E. (2002). A quantitative review of prospective evidence linking psychosocial factors with hypertension development. *Psychosomatic Medicine, 64*, 758–766.

Shavit, Y., et al. (1985). Stress, opioid peptides, the immune system and cancer. *Journal of Immunology, 135*, 834–837.

Sheps, D.S., et al. (2002). Mental stress induced ischemia and all cause mortality in persons with coronary artery disease: Results in the psychophysiological investigations of myocardial ischemia study. *Circulation, 84*, 1780–1789.

Siegman, A. (2000). Antagonistic behavior, dominance, hostility, and coronary heart disease. *Psychosomatic Medicine*. *62*, 248–257.

Smith, R. W., et al. (2002). Psychosocial influences on the development and course of coronary heart disease: Current status and implications for practice and research. *Journal of Consulting and Clinical Psychology, 70*, 548–568.

Spiegel, D., & Giese-Davis, J. (2003). Depression and cancer: Mechanisms and disease progression. *Biological Psychiatry,* 545, 269–282.

Spira, M., & Carlon, L. (2000). *Psychosomatic Medicine,* 62–65.

Stolbach, L. (2003). Does fighting spirit improve medical outcomes of cancer patients? *Advances, 19,* 17–18.

Stoney, C.M., West, S.G., & Hudges, J.W. (2002). Acute psychological stress reduces plasma triglyceride clearance. *Psychophysiology, 39,* 80–85.

Surwit, R. (2004). *The Mind-Body Diabetes Revolution.* New York: Free Press.

Theorell, T. (2005). Coping with critical life events and lack of control: The exertion of control. *Psychoneuroendocrinology , 30,* 1027–1032.

Van Melle, J.P., de Jonge, P., et al. (2004). Prognostic association for depression following myocardial infarction with mortality and cardiovascular events: A meta-analysis. *Psychosomatic Medicine, 66,* 814–882.

Wassertheil-Smoller, S. (2004). Depression and cardiovascular sequelae in postmenopausal women. *Archives of Internal Medicine, 164,* 289–298.

Watson, M. (1996). Adaptational style and dispositional structure: coping in the context of the five-factor model. *Journal of Personality,* 64:737.

Williams, J.E., Paton, L.C., & Sieglar, I.C. (2000). Anger proneness predicts coronary heart disease risk. *Circulation, 101,* 2034–2039.

Yan, L.L., et al. (2003). Psychosocial factors and risk of hypertension: The coronary artery and risk development study in young adults (Cardia) study. *Journal of the American Medical Association, 22,* 2136–2148.

Zutra, A., et al (1989). Life stress and lymphocyte alterations among patients with rheumatoid arthritis. *Health Psychology, 8,* 1–14.

D. EXERCISES

Match the following psychosocial phenomena with the appropriate health or illness:

A *fighting spirit* is associated with

____

____

Social support has been associated with (name two)

____

____

Hostility is associated with

____

____

Anger, anxiety, depression are associated with

Depression can also be associated with

Optimism is associated with

High stress is associated with (name three problems)

Answer the following questions using material from this chapter:

1. You are seeing a patient with cancer. This disease is associated with a compromised immune system. Which two psychosocial phenomena might help this person?

2. Patients feel better, survive longer, and have fewer days of debilitation when they express what kind of "spirit"?

3. Healthful blood pressure is associated with what psychosocial phenomena?

4. Name three maladies associated with stress.

____

____

5. Hypertension is associated with what psychosocial phenomena?

____

____

6. Name three maladies associated with depression.

____

____

7. A suppressed immune system is associated with which psychosocial phenomena?

____

____

8. Those who manage their anger in a constructive manner are likely to have lower ____________________?

9. A patient who is experiencing slower-than-normal wound healing is likely to be experiencing which psychosocial phenomena?

____

____

10. In working with hypertensive patients, which psychosocial phenomena should you consider helping them to change?

____

____

Apply information learned in this chapter to the following case by isolating the psychosocial phenomena in this woman's life that might be associated with her condition. Check your answers against the Answer Guide. Then, challenge yourself to say how/why these might be significant.

Client Situation

You are working with a woman recently diagnosed with breast cancer. She is otherwise in good health but lives alone and has few "real" friends. You realize that she has more down days than up (is she losing her optimism?), and she often remarks that she "contributes little to her world." Her work as a nurse requires much responsibility, but she perceives that she has little power to do what she feels is correct. Sometime, she feels what she describes as "overly angry."

Answer Guide to the Case

1. First, the woman lives alone and has few real friends. She lacks social support, which could lower her immunity; you know from the chapter that there is reasonable evidence that social support could extend life expectancy in breast cancer victims.
2. Second, she has many down days and feels she contributes little; you perceive her as losing optimism. If she becomes depressed, then she may be more likely to compromise her immune system.
3. Third, she is in a high-demand job with little power. This is a possible cause of stress. How might stress influence her health?
4. Fourth, she tells you about her anger. What role might anger play in her situation?

5

Mechanisms of Stress

Many studies in the scientific literature demonstrate the role of distress in illness. In fact, one recent report estimates that 85% of visits to a physician are for stress-related aliments and complaints (Cleveland Clinic, 2002). As you learned in Chapter 4, the person under constant distress is vulnerable to several illnesses. This seems to be due to the secretion of hormones different from the person not under this stress. The secretion of these hormones (e.g., cortisol) has been associated with physical disease (e.g., atherosclerosis). Distress also affects the immune system, resulting in fewer lymphocytes. The person under distress is more subject to infections than the person not under distress. Because distress seems to play a key role in health and illness, we devote this chapter to giving you an opportunity to increase your knowledge of the phenomenon of stress.

A. GOALS

1. To understand the dynamics of stress.
2. To understand how stress might affect health.
3. To better understand what might contribute to stress in your life.
4. To appreciate ways to manage stress.

B. LEARNING OBJECTIVES

After working through this chapter, you will be able to

1. List physical factors involved in stress.
2. List at least five ways stress could affect health.
3. List the stress producers in your life.
4. Apply at least one way to prevent stress.
5. Apply at least one way to manage stress.

C. INFORMATION GUIDE

In this chapter, we present an overview of stress. Our purpose is to keep it simple with a view to applying the information in a clinical situation. However, stress is such an important psychosocial phenomenon in MindBody medicine that we include a more detailed discussion of stress in Appendix C.

1. Nature of stress
   a. Definitions:
      Stress is a physical, chemical, or an emotional factor that causes bodily or mental tension and may be a factor in disease causation (*Merriam-Webster Medical Dictionary*).
      Hans Selye, the classic researcher on stress defines stress as "nonspecific response of the body to any demand" (1980).
   b. What are the things that might cause stress (i.e., *stressors*)? Stressors can be internal or external factors or stimuli that produce stress. Stressors may be physical, biological, environmental, situational, and spiritual, whatever meaning a person attributes to his or her spirituality.
   c. Dynamics of stress: A phenomenon (e.g., event, memory, emotion) is perceived as a threat. This perception initiates the production of corticotropin-releasing factor by the hypothalamus. Corticotropin-releasing factor acts on the pituitary gland, which in turn secretes adrenocorticotropic hormone, releasing a cascade of other hormones (e.g., norepinephrine, epinephrine, and glucocorticoids).
   d. Types of stress: Technically, there are two types of stress: distress and eustress.
      Distress: This type of stress is perceived as overwhelming. Although research reports do not always specify, distress seems to be the experience that is detrimental to our health and is usually referred to in the research as stress. In distress, we perceive the situation or event as confused and hopeless, and that there is no way to change. An example of this type of stress would be found in an abusive marriage or job situation that is difficult to leave: The person perceives and believes that he or she is trapped.
      Eustress: This type of stress is rousing and challenging but manageable. It results in significant elevation of serum catecholamines (e.g., norepinephrine, epinephrine, dopamine) with no change in serum prolactin or cortisol concentrations. In eustress, we perceive the event or situation as an opportunity, and there is a sense of hope, such as an exciting but challenging job situation: We have options.
2. Causes of stress: internal and external
   a. *Internal* or "subjective" stress: Most stress is caused by MindBody interaction, for example, how we perceive a situation, what we

believe about it, and what we tell ourselves (e.g., if we perceive the animal in the pasture to be a bull, we believe it is a bull, and we tell ourselves we are in danger as it comes toward us, then we will have a stress reaction; this happens even though the animal is a gentle cow).

b. *External* or "objective" stress: Certain events have been seen as stressors. For example, the death of a spouse, divorce, marital separation, jail term, death of a family member, personal injury or illness, being fired from work, and even something that could be a happy event like marriage carries with it stress (hopefully without feelings of being trapped). Remember, in both internal and external stress the vital element is whether one perceives and believes there is hope (eustress) or no hope (distress).

3. Recognizing your stress: Stress may be a challenge to recognize and differentiate from depression. In clinical situations, patients who are depressed will often be sad and feel down, whereas the person under stress will usually not feel sadness but rather tension, irritability, and a sense of urgency and believe they "can't stop." To help you recognize stress, discover whether the person is experiencing objective stress such as a death of a loved one and how they interpret the situation (subjective stress), whether the situation is an objective stressor or not. So, in summary if you are perceiving that you have unmet demands placed on you, you feel nervous and tense, you cannot stop to take a break, and you experience sleeplessness because of concern about problems, then you are probably experiencing stress.
4. Stress prevention and management: To help prevent stress and manage it when it does occur, there are definite proactive approaches. The following is a list of some of these approaches:

Meditation: This is the basic daily training to help us be ready for the assaults of stress (Miller, Fletcher, et al., 1995; Ospina-Kammerer & Figley, 2003). Meditation is like weight training to the athlete; it makes one ready.

Exercise: Like meditation, exercise makes us ready to face the stressors of life. It also tends to minimize stress if stress occurs. Any type of physical exercise will almost always help with stress. Make sure you are in proper physical shape to exercise, and that whatever you do is done properly and at the correct time and place and with proper equipment. Also, remember that if you have a panic disorder, vigorous exercise may initially exacerbate it so you must start your exercise program gradually and slowly.

Organization: Lack of organization results in frustrations and a sense of helplessness and stress. A sure way for most people to be stressed is to have a cluttered environment, conflicting schedules, and lack of any form of stress reduction in daily life. Know your time limits and stick within them and arrange your space and time in such a way that a you have ease in locating objects and knowing where you should be according to your schedule of events.

Rehearsal: Unpreparedness gives a sense of vulnerability and lack of control. Again, stress is the result. Plan ahead, know what you will do or say, and be prepared for surprises. These behaviors will make you feel comfortable about what happens.

Practice positive self-statements: As you work with patients, you will discover how often they participate in heightening their stress by what they say to themselves. If you are experiencing stress, then you might notice that you also practice "negative self talk." Your self-talk may be contributing to your stress. These self-statements are not positive (self-enhancing) but negative (self-limiting). For example, you will hear someone make statements such as: "I can't" or "I never can." By simply changing some of this limiting talk, you will begin to perceive a sense of control in your life, and this sense of control will alleviate some stress. As an example of helping in this area, you might stop repeating a statement of necessity such as "I can't do something." In place of these limiting statements, substitute a more freeing statement like "'until now, it has been difficult." This simple change in self-talk helps eliminate the stressful limitations of 'I can't." With "until now," there is at least the possibility of change and therefore less sense of limitation, frustration, and stress.

Reframe the situation: Note and focus on any positive aspects of a situation and emphasize the positive. This is not always an easy intervention but here are two examples to help you understand it more clearly:

Some illnesses, believe it or not, can be seen to have a positive impact on a person's life. Often, the person who has received a diagnosis of diabetes will be able to do much to bring about health through a change of lifestyle. This change might consist of a healthy diet, better and regular exercise, smoking cessation, and activities to lower stress and increase social support. In working with this person with diabetes, the *reframe* helps them to understand that even though they are experiencing an illness, there are valuable things they have control over that can make life better; hence, you reframe the situation from just being sick to the positive possibilities of a better and longer life.

Another example is often found in working with patients experiencing agoraphobia with panic (a condition in which a person is overafraid to go outside the home); the patient will relate that he/she has the ability to leave the home only twice during the week. Typically, the patient overlooks the positive event of the ability to leave the home at all. When you emphasize this event and what it accomplished, you are emphasizing a positive aspect of the patient's life, a type of reframing.

Assertiveness training: Often, stress is a product of a sense of lack of power. When we do not know how to be appropriately assertive, we feel that lack of power. Simply training patients to say "No," to make appropriate requests of others, and to be comfortable in doing so often is a major step in lowering stress.

Laugh: Look for the humor in situations, read or view funny stories, or practice telling yourself jokes. This is a solid stress reliever.

SUGGESTED READING

American Academy of Family Physicians. (1998). *Facts About Family Practice.* Kansas City, MO: American Academy of Family Physicians. [This is a useful reference for anyone interested in working with physicians.]

Antoni, M.H. (1993). Stress management: Strategies that work. In D. Goleman & J. Gurin (Eds.), *Mind Body Medicine* (pp. 385–401). Yonkers, NY: Consumer Reports Books. [This is a good collection of procedures to help in stress management.]

Arnetz, B.B. (1991). White collar stress: What studies of physicians can teach us. *Psychotherapy Psychosomatic, 55,* 197–200.

Breznitz, S., & Goldberger, L. (1993). *Stress Research at a Crossroads.* New York: Free Press.

Buckingham, J.C., Gillies, G.E., & Cowell, A. (1997). *Stress, Stress Hormones and the Immune System.* New York: Wiley.

Carroll, J.F.X., & White, W.L. (1982). Theory building: Integrating individual and environmental factors within an ecological framework. In W. S. Paine (Ed.), *Job Stress and Burnout* (pp. 41–61). Beverly Hills, CA: Sage.

Cunningham, A.J. (1981). Mind, body and immune response. In Ader, R. (Ed.). *Psychoneuroimmunology* (pp. 609–616). Orlando, FL: Academic Press.

Figley, C. (1995). *Compassion Fatigue.* New York: Brunner/Mazel.

Figley, C. (1998). *Burnout in Families.* Boca Raton, FL: CRC Press.

Figley, C.R., & Kleber, R.J. (1995). Beyond the victim: Secondary traumatic stress. In R. J. Kleber, C. R. Figley, & P. R. Gersons (Eds.), *Beyond Trauma* (pp. 76–95). New York: Plenum Press.

Goleman, D., & Gurin, J. (1993). *Mind Body Medicine.* Yonkers, NY: Consumer Union.

Kiecolt-Glaser, J.K., & Glaser, R. (1993). Mind and immunity. In D. Goleman & J. Gurin (Eds.), *Mind Body Medicine* (pp. 19–39). Yonkers, NY: Consumer Reports Books.

Kiecolt-Glaser, J.K., & Marucha, P.T. (1995). Slowing of wound healing by psychological stress. *Lancet, 346,* 1194–1196.

Kiecolt-Glaser, et al. (1998). Marital stress: Immunologic, neuroendocrine, and autonomic correlates. *Annals of the New York Academy of Science, 840,* 656–666. [The Kiecolt-Glasers are pioneer researchers in the field of stress. We can recommend each of their works.]

Kugelman, R. (1992). *Stress: The Nature and History of Engineered Grief.* Westport, CT: Praeger.

Lovallo, W.R. (1997). *Stress and Health.* Thousand Oaks, CA: Sage.

McEwen, B.S. (1993). Stress and the individual mechanisms leading to disease. *Archives of Internal Medicine, 153*, 2093–2101.

Miller, J., Fletcher, K., et al. (1995) Three-year follow-up and clinical implications of a mindfulness meditation-based stress reduction intervention in the treatment of anxiety disorders. *General Hospital Psychiatry, 17*, 192–200.

Ospina-Kammerer, V., & Figley, C. (2003) An evaluation of the Respiratory One Method (ROM) in reducing emotional exhaustion among family physician residents. *International Journal of Emergency Mental Health, 5*, (1).

Schafer, W. (1996). *Stress Management for Wellness.* Fort Worth, TX: Harcourt Brace College Publishers.

Selye, H. (1936). *The Stress of Life.* New York: McGraw-Hill.

Selye, H. (1980). *Seyle's Guide to Stress Research.* New York: Van Nostrand Reinhold. [Dr. Selye is the classic thinker in this area. His works are worth referencing for anyone interested in a deeper understanding of stress.]

Solomon, F.G. (1997). Clinical and social implications of stress-induced neuroendocrine-immune interactions. In J. C. Buckingham, G. E. Gillies, & A. M. Cowell (Eds.), *Stress, Stress Hormones and the Immune System* (pp. 385–401). New York: Wiley.

Spiegel, D. (1999). Healing words: Emotional expression and disease outcome. *Journal of the American Medical Association, 281*, 1328–1329.

D. EXERCISES

1. Commit to memory a definition of stress with examples.

2. Commit to memory an outline of the dynamics of stress.

3. Identify and list possible stresses in your life.

4. Learn two stress management tools.

5. Learn two stress prevention tools.

6. Review Appendix C for further information and understanding of stress.

6

Physical Systems That Relate to MindBody Medicine

In the previous chapters, you gained insight into what the mind does: mental activities. You studied the interventions that influence these mental activities. Further, you considered the psychosocial phenomena that relate to our health and mental activities and how they relate to stress. All this information (i.e., mental activities, MindBody interventions, psychosocial phenomena, and stress) needs to be considered in relation to the physical self of a person. This physical self is composed of various body systems. Our focus in this chapter is on the key body systems involved in MindBody medicine. In this chapter, we consider answers to the following questions: What are these systems? How do they function?

It is likely that all body systems are involved, but three systems are prominent in the research: nervous, immune, and endocrine systems. In this chapter, we also focus on these three body systems and give you an overview of each. We include illustrations of how MindBody medicine interventions might influence the system. Remember that this is a model to help you think in terms of influencing a system in a particular way. Much valid research is needed to establish more confidence that a particular intervention will work in a way we currently believe it does. The hypothesis presented here is that particular MindBody interventions may influence a body system in such a way that the system changes for a healthier function. In knowing something of the system, you can more accurately apply a specific MindBody technique to influence that system. We have included examples to help you. Some of these reflect current usage in MindBody medicine (consult Chapter 1 and Appendix A); others are speculative based on our understanding of the system and the intervention. As research improves, you will be better able to apply a specific, well-researched intervention to achieve a definite result with a specific system.

The Exercise section gives you more opportunity to practice and enhance your understanding. You will deepen your understanding of these systems and how to apply MindBody interventions as you appreciate the working of the particular system (e.g., if you know that the sympathetic nervous system increases heart rate, then you can apply a specific MindBody intervention to turn that system "on" or "off" deliberately, depending on whether you desire increased heart rate). As you deepen your understanding of these systems, you will realize how they are affected by activities of the mind and how specific interventions might affect a system.

As you study each body system, think about how you might apply information learned from former chapters. Be speculative and creative. Think how a particular way a person thinks (mental functions) might affect a body system. Think how an intervention might be employed to influence that thinking and thus the body system's function. This thought process is the focus for now, not the correct intervention (remember research results are still mixed on many interventions, but as you think accurately in applying MindBody medicine then you become facile in applying the most scientific approach as it is discovered). Focus on answering the following questions:

1. Which mental activity might be involved in influencing the system?
2. Which MindBody intervention might be employed to influence that mental activity to strengthen or inhibit that system for health?

The following examples will help:

1. A mental activity that relates to a body system may be *belief*. If a person believes he or she is in danger, then often that person will have a sympathetic nervous response. This response is based more on the mental activity (belief) than on the objective reality. Perhaps this belief could be changed via imagery, thereby changing the response from sympathetic to parasympathetic.
2. Another mind activity is *imagination*. There is evidence that some people can use their imagination to enhance the immune system. If you are working with a patient whose problem is immune weakness (e.g., cancer, AIDS), perhaps the employment of imaging B cells and T cells becoming stronger or increasing in number would be helpful. Perhaps a MindBody intervention to assist this particular patient to use imagery would be to employ hypnosis.
3. *Perception* is a common mental activity that relates to illness. This is often evident in working with patients who experience pain. The pain is increased when the patient perceives that the pain indicates a deadly problem. Intervening to change the patient's perception will help manage the pain. Cognitive-behavioral therapy may be a good choice to assist the patient in changing this perception.

Be aware that this chapter is an introduction. Depending on your background in anatomy and physiology, you will need more or less time devoted to this chapter. It is merely a beginning. As you become involved in MindBody medicine, you will need to deepen your knowledge of these body systems, possibly other systems, and the pathophysiology of specific diseases.

A. GOALS

1. To deepen your understanding of the body systems involved in MindBody medicine.
2. To lay a foundation for targeting specific interventions to specific body systems.
3. To understand better how the functions of these systems relate to health and illness.

B. LEARNING OBJECTIVES

After working through this chapter, you will be able to

1. Give from memory a definition of each body system discussed.
2. Give an example of a possible MindBody intervention for each system.

C. INFORMATION GUIDE

It is likely that all body systems are involved in MindBody medicine. In this chapter, we focus on the three most referenced in the literature: the nervous, immune, and endocrine systems. Keep in mind that these systems are interconnected, and that by influencing one it is likely that we influence others. This fact is the basis for psychoneuorimmunology, a term you have likely come across in your study of MindBody medicine. Both Robert Ader and the Glasers have helped us by listing some examples of this interconnection (Ader, 1990; Goleman & Gurin, 1993). Here is a synopsis of their thoughts:

- Changes in the central nervous system (CNS) alter immune responses, and an immune response alters central nervous system activity.
- Changes in hormone and neurotransmitter levels alter immune responses and vice versa.
- Lymphocytes are chemically responsive to hormones and neurotransmitters.
- Immunologic activity can be modified by classical conditioning.

1. Nervous System

The nervous system, along with the endocrine system, provides most of the control of your body. It can be divided into the central nervous system (CNS), the peripheral nervous system (PNS), and the autonomous nervous system (ANS).

Central Nervous System

Microlevel. The *neuron* is the basic microlevel instrument for transporting information such as beliefs and self-talk. Neurons are the basic functional unit of the nervous systems. There are over 100 million neurons in the CNS. Figure 6.1 depicts how a neuron might look. Impulses travel from the dendrites to the presynaptic terminals. At this juncture, the impulses go across the synaptic cleft, to the postsynaptic terminal, to the dendrite of another neuron. Synapses help control some kinds of information flow, particularly muscle contractions. The large part of information from the brain is kept straight, not by close physical proximity of the system, but rather by the specificity of the receptors (Pert, 2002).

Macrolevel The brain and spinal cord make up the macrolevel of the CNS. Figure 6.2 will help you locate important areas of this system.

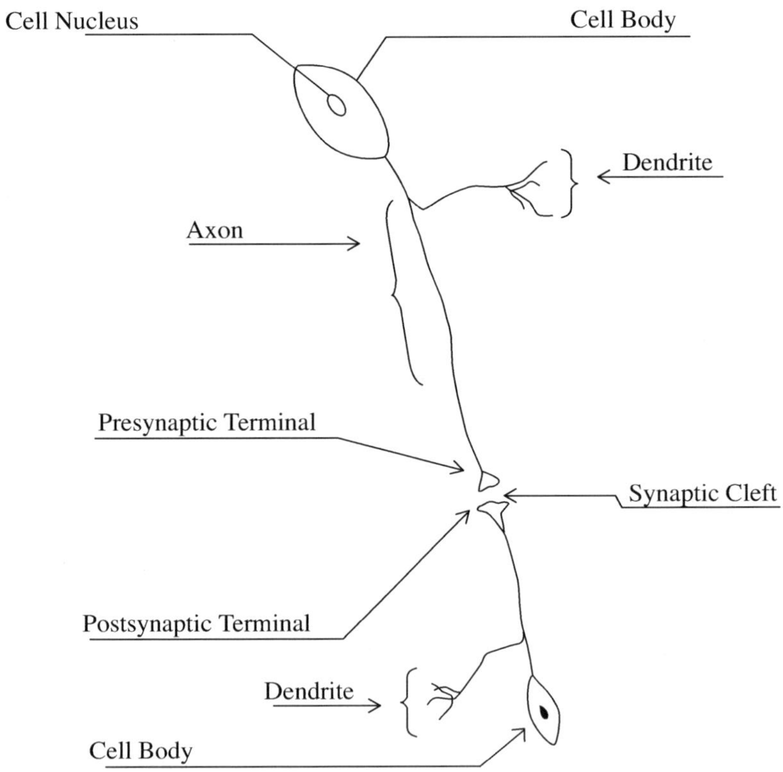

FIGURE 6.1. Schematic of a neuron.

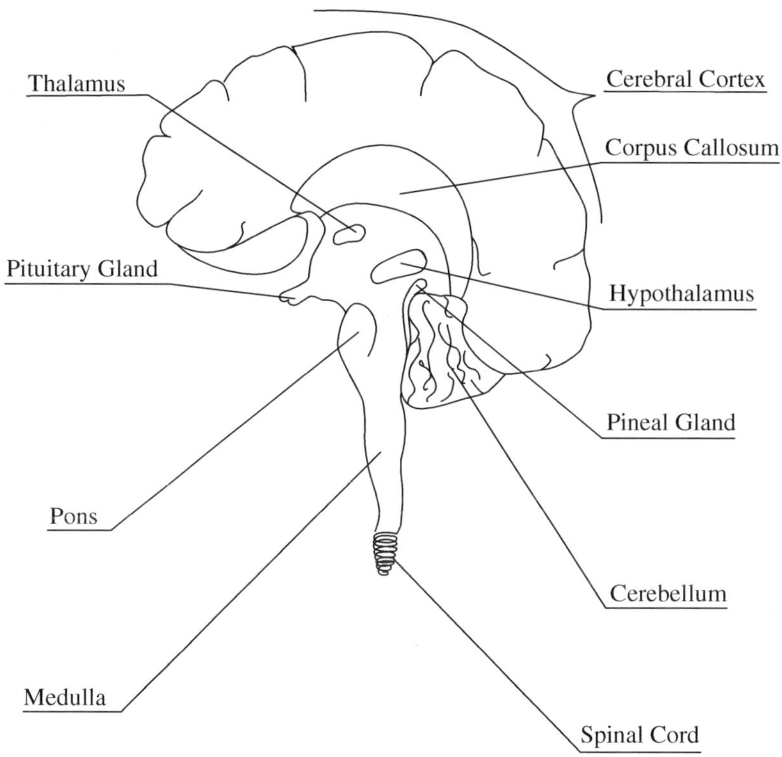

FIGURE 6.2 Schematic of the brain (cerebrum).

Some known functions of the six main parts of the CNS are as follows:

- The *spinal cord* controls movement of the limbs and the trunk. It receives and processes information from the skin, joints, and muscles of the limbs.
- The *medulla oblongata* lies directly above the spinal cord and includes several centers responsible for such vital autonomic functions as digestion, breathing, and the control of heart rate.
- The *pons*, which lies above the medulla, conveys information from the cerebral hemisphere to the cerebellum.
- The *cerebellum* lies behind the pons and is connected to the brain stem by several major fiber tracts called *peduncles*. The cerebellum modulates the force and range of movement and is involved in the learning of motor skills.
- The *cerebral cortex* is the extensive outer layer of gray tissue of the cerebral hemispheres and is largely responsible for the nervous functions.
- The *thalamus* relays sensory stimuli to the cerebral cortex and integrative functions.
- The *pituitary gland* stores and releases hormones.

- The *pineal gland* (or *pineal body*) secretes melatonin.
- The *diencephalon* lies rostral to the midbrain and contains two structures. One, the *thalamus*, processes most of the information reaching the cerebral cortex from the rest of the CNS. The other, the *hypothalamus*, regulates autonomic, endocrine, and visceral functions.

Application of MindBody Medicine Using Knowledge of the Central Nervous System

You are helping a patient who suffers from a brain tumor. By understanding more clearly where the tumor is located in the brain (the anatomy) and what that area controls (the physiology), you might better help the patient with an intervention.

The tumor is in the cerebellum. There is some evidence that some people (we do not yet know the distinguishing variables) can employ imagery to shrink tumors (Dossey, 1999). You instruct your patient in using the MindBody intervention of visual imagery. By your understanding of the location and function of the cerebellum, you help the patient create an image of having full range of movement and motor skills (you have used your knowledge of both anatomy and physiology). The mental activities affected are belief, perception (the patient perceives and believes that the method will help), and imagination (the patient uses her imagination to create the picture of the tumor shrinking).

Your patient's condition is associated with a bleed in the cerebral cortex. The patient's family expresses a strong faith in prayer and tells you that there is also a prayer group at their church. You know that prayer seems to help in cardiac surgery, AIDS, pregnancy, and rheumatoid arthritis. Even though there is no evidence that prayer would help control the bleeding, there is also no known harm in its use in this situation (of course, all known interventions are also employed). Might the prayer intervention be more effective by your use of your understanding the anatomy of where the bleed is located in the cerebral cortex and counseling the family to envision this area as they pray?

Peripheral Nervous System. The PNS provides a complete network of motor and sensory fibers connecting the CNS to the rest of the body. Pairs of nerves enter and exit the spinal cord between each vertebra. Branches of these nerves are responsible for sensation and motion throughout the body. In addition, there are 12 pairs of cranial nerves that travel between the head and neck without passing through the spinal cord.

Autonomic Nervous System. The brain influences health and healing through a special group of nerves that connects the physiological control center of the brain with virtually all of the body's tissues and organs. This group of nerves, the ANS, regulates glands, smooth muscle, and cardiac muscle.

The ANS has two divisions, the *sympathetic* and the *parasympathetic*. In the broadest terms, these two sets of nerves tend to work in opposition to each other on various body functions. (For example, sympathetic activity tends to increase heart rate; parasympathetic activity tends to reduce it. Sympathetic activity tends to decrease digestive activity, and parasympathetic activity tends to increase it.)

The autonomic nervous system derives its name from the fact that the activities of both the sympathetic and the parasympathetic nerves normally operate without conscious control. In other words, you do not have to think about how fast you want to breathe or how fast your heart should beat. You do not consciously direct the minute-to-minute digestion of your dinner. Control over the internal organs is relatively automatic. Built-in mechanisms in the brain maintain homeostasis (Guyton, 1991).

The sympathetic nervous system stimulates alarm. This process releases epinephrine and norepinephrine from the adrenal medulla. When the sympathetic nervous system is active, the body usually reacts in the following ways:

- Pupils dilate.
- Lachrymal glands decrease output.
- Salivary glands increase output.
- Heart rate increases; strength of heart contractions increases.
- Blood goes to the mesenteric region.
- Respiratory passages open.
- Stomach contractions and digestive secretions are inhibited.
- Intestinal peristalsis is inhibited.
- The bladder relaxes.

The parasympathetic nervous system brings about relaxation. This process releases acetylcholine (a neurotransmitter). When the parasympathetic nervous system is active, the body usually reacts in the following ways:

- Pupils constrict.
- Heart rate decreases.
- Respiratory passages constrict.
- The stomach contracts; digestive fluids are secreted.
- Intestinal peristalsis increases.
- The bladder contracts.
- Erection occurs.

Application of MindBody Medicine Using Your Knowledge of the Autonomic Nervous System

Illustration 1

A patient informs you that his panic is increased when he feels his heart rate increased (sympathetic nervous response). You know that evoking the parasympathetic system will result in a decrease in heart rate. Whether the increase in heart rate causes panic is a result of panic or is concomitant with the panic, by regulating the rate you may be able to help abort a panic attack. Therefore, to help the patient achieve a parasympathetic state you teach him meditation for a daily routine and a short yoga breathing technique for when he finds himself in a situation of potential panic. The MindBody interventions are meditation and yoga to focus on bringing about parasympathetic nervous response; the mental activities affected are possibly the patient's perception (changed from perceiving that he has "no power" in this situation to having "a plan"); belief (he believes that your suggestions will work, and that he now has some control); and memory (he remembers that he has been able to change the situation in the past). Your knowledge of the autonomic nervous system was an asset in your accurate intervention.

Illustration 2

Your patient tells you that he will be taking a beta-blocker for his hypertension. He feels week and dizzy on some occasions. His physician informed him that this might occur with the medication, and that part of what is happening is a slowing of his heart rate. He is requesting your help to employ MindBody medicine. After you consult with his physician to obtain complete understanding of the pathophysiology of your patient's condition, you help the patient develop a visual imaging exercise by which he envisions himself running vigorously, and this helps restore his heart rate to normal.

2. The Immune System

The immune system protects the body (you) from the invasion of foreign pathogens (i.e., viruses, bacteria, fungi, and parasites). Also, the immune system can detect and eliminate cells that have become damaged (e.g., neoplastically transformed). This system is both innate (i.e., present from birth) and acquired (i.e., developed as a result of encountering new substances, e.g., bacteria).

We present an overview of the acquired immune system. This system seems most affected by mental activity (e.g., stress). Consult Table 6.1 for a scheme of immune system entities and their relationship to each other. This will assist you as we review the system.

Overview of Immune System

Myeloid Progeneration

1. Granulocytes: These are large granules in cytoplasm.
    - The neutrophils have a lysosome filled with proteolytic enzymes that digest bacteria and other invaders. They are increased in

TABLE 6.1
Key Elements of the Immune System

Bone Marrow Produces Pluripotent Stem Cells That Develop Into		
Myeloid Progeneration Cells		Lymphoid Progeneration Cells
Types		Types
Granulocytes	Monocytes (which differentiate to macrophages)	T Cells (from Thymus Gland)
a. Neutrophils		NK cells (natural killer cells)
b. Eosinophils		B cells (stimulated by T-cells, which develop into plasma cells)
c. Basophils (which differentiate to mass cells)		

number when infections start. They play the primary role in inflammation, easily recognizing foreign antigens and destroying them through phagocytosis (the engulfing of these cells by the neutrophil to kill the engulfed cell). Neutrophils may overreact to stimuli and become involved in tissue destruction (e.g., rheumatoid arthritis, myocardial reperfusion injury, respiratory distress syndrome, and ulcerative colitis).

- Eosinophils increase with allergic reaction and are known to destroy parasitic organisms.
- Basophils have a role that is not completely clear, but they are involved in inflammatory processes.

2. Monocytes are also phagocytes: They develop into macrophages when they leave the bloodstream. Their lysosome contains lipase, which digests the thick lipid membranes possessed by some bacteria.

Lymphoid Progeneration

Lymphocytes are the white blood cells that help protect us from invaders. Lymphocytes are either B cells (humoral), T cells (cellular), or natural killer (NK) cells.

B cells (humoral) protect us by producing antibodies (tiny proteins that help to fight infection). These antibodies are built to recognize specific invaders and antigens (this is a substance, usually a protein, on the surface of a cell or bacterium that stimulates the production of an antibody). These B-cell antibodies connect with the antigen and expose part of it so that it is recognized as an invader by a helper T cell. The helper T cell attaches to the B cells and releases interleukins, which stimulate the B cell to become an antibody factor (called a *plasma cell*), which in turn pumps millions of identical antibodies into the bloodstream to hunt down invading antigens.

T cells (cellular) do not produce antibodies. The T cells circulate constantly throughout the body, ready to assist the B cells.

NK cells are large granular lymphocytes that bond to cells and engulf them by releasing cytotoxin. They are necessary for the natural immune response.

Dysfunction of the Immune System

The wonderful immune system that protects us is also often part of the process of illness. The system can become too weak to help fight off an invader (is underactive); it can become so powerful that it overwhelms us (is hyperactive); or it can turn on us, attacking our organs as if they were the invading dangerous organism (is misdirected). In appreciating the manner in which the immune system becomes a problem rather than a help, we may be able to tailor our MindBody interventions to focus on the appropriate need (e.g., if we know that the immune system has become too weak to protect us, then we can tailor an intervention to strengthen it). The following illustrations of the dysfunctional immune system will help you appreciate this. Be aware that the examples used in the illustrations are to help you understand the process of application and are not definitive guidelines of interventions. As we cautioned in the Introduction, much MindBody medicine is still in the basic stage of scientific research. One of the challenges faced in application is that a particular intervention may work well with a particular person under a specific set of circumstances but be difficult to repeat in others.

There are three ways the system can be dysfunctional: by underactivity, hyperactivity, or misdirected activity.

Underactivity

In underactivity, the immune system lacks the rigor or number of cells required to protect the body. Some illnesses associated with underactivity are as follows:

Cancer
AIDS
Hepatitis

Application of MindBody Medicine

You learned from Chapters 4 and 5 that stress lowers the immune system's ability to protect us. Reducing stress by helping a patient change his or her perception and belief about a potentially stressful situation may be helpful in improving the immune system or at least keeping that system from becoming weaker. Many interventions seem to bring about the relaxation response (Chapter 1). Two that will likely help protect from stress are visual imagery and positive self talk.

Imagery combined with hypnosis is a potentially powerful MindBody intervention. You could apply this information in working with any condition that is associated with underactive immunity. Thus, the patient experiencing AIDS might be helped by envisioning their B, T, and NK cells becoming stronger and more actively attacking the invading virus.

Hyperactivity

A hyperactive immune system overwhelms a body system, usually because of the overproduction of defenders (e.g., leukocytes). Some illnesses associated with hyperactivity are as follows:

- Idiopathic thrombocytopenia
- Asthma
- Allergies

Application of MindBody Medicine

Since illnesses associated with hyperactive immunity might be helped by toning down the immune response, you could focus an intervention on doing just that, perhaps by using hypnosis with music and imagery. The imagery could focus on the immune cells quieting and becoming normally active rather than hyperactive. The hypnosis and music would assist in achieving a needed level of concentration.

You are working with a patient who experiences asthma. From what you have learned in Chapter 1, you could assist the patient in employing group support and expressive writing as there is some evidence that these interventions in some way help modify this condition.

Misdirected Immune System

The misdirected immune system attacks the self (autoimmunity). Some illnesses resulting from misdirected immune system are as follows:

- Rheumatoid arthritis: The immune system acts as if there is an infection within the joint, producing enzymes that attack and eat away at cartilage
- Spondylitis
- Type I diabetes: The immune cells system destroys insulin production
- Systemic lupus erythematosus
- Glomerulonephritis
- Rheumatic fever
- Polymyositis
- Autoimmune thyroiditis

Autoimmune hemolytic anemia
Idiopathic thrombocytopenic purpura
Myasthenia gravis
Scleroderma
Sjogren syndrome
Vasculitis

Application of MindBody Medicine

The literature reports MindBody interventions for these diseases (Smyth, 1999). However, the exact mechanism is not as clear as for the hyperactive and underactive immune problems. That is, we do not know whether a particular intervention (e.g., expressive writing) affects stress levels or in some way directly refocuses the immune activity away from the host. We might, however, theorize that an intervention aimed at redirecting the immune system would be worth considering. For example, a patient with rheumatoid arthritis is helped to achieve a deep hypnotic trance. During the trance, suggestion and imagery are developed that focus on the immune system "backing off" from the self and functioning normally.

This illustration focuses on changing the mechanism of a misdirected immune system. Actual research on the individual diseases is rarer. Most of the reliable material to date focuses on rheumatoid arthritis. The interventions that seem to help are support groups, expressive writing, and prayer.

3. *Endocrine System*

The endocrine system consists of ductless glands that secrete hormones directly into the bloodstream (e.g., pancreas secretes insulin, adrenal glands secrete adrenalin, etc.).

Hormones are chemical substances secreted into the body by one cell or a group of cells, and they exercise a physiological control over other cells of the body.

At this time, there is very little research on manipulating the endocrine system using MindBody intervention. Nevertheless, it is a reasonable hypothesis that we could direct or strengthen, similar to the manner used for the immune system, hormones to perform their function by employing MindBody interventions. Thus, you might employ visual imagery of appropriate hormones behaving in a healthful manner by training the patient to employ this visualization after the patient meditates.

SUGGESTED READING

Ader, R. (1990). *Psychoneuroimmunology*. San Diego, CA: Academic Press.
Ader might be considered the "father" of psychoneuroimmunology. His original research set the stage for much of the thinking in MindBody medicine.

Black, P.H. (1994). Psychoneuroendocrinology of stress and its immune consequences. *Antimicrobe Agents Chemotherapy, 38,* 1–6.

Connolly, K. (2004). *Brain activity and the development of posttraumatic stress disorder.* Unpublished research paper, Florida State University, College of Social Work.

Dossey, L. (1999). *Reinventing Medicine.* San Francisco: Harper. Dr. Dossey puts forth interesting examples and thought-provoking ideas. [This is a book that will enhance the ability of readers to think outside the box.]

Goleman, D., & Gurin, J. (1993). *Mind Body Medicine.* New York: Consumer Reports Books.

Guyton, A. (1991). *Textbook of Medical Physiology.* New York: Saunders. [A basic and well-done text to better understand this subject.]

Pert, C. (2002). The wisdom of the receptors: Neuropeptides, the emotions, and bodymind. *Advances, 18,* 30–34. [Dr. Pert's thoughts will stimulate the reader to review the usual view of the mind.]

Pliszka, S. (2003). *Neuroscience for the Mental Health Clinician.* New York: Guilford Press.

Smith, R.S. (1991). The immune system is a key factor in the etiology of psychosocial disease. *Medical Hypnosis, 34,* 49–57.

Smyth, J.M., (1999). Effects of writing about stressful experiences on symptom reduction in patients with asthma and rheumatoid arthritis. A randomized trial. *JAMA, 281,* 1304–1309.

D. EXERCISES

1. Define from memory the

   Central nervous system
   Peripheral nervous system
   Autonomic nervous system
   Immune system and include hyperimmunity, hypoimmunity, and misdirected
   Endocrine system
2. Practice applying MindBody medicine to the following examples (refer to Chapter 1 and Appendix B for help in choosing specific interventions):

Case 1

Your patient has cancer. Do you want to help her strengthen, redirect, or weaken her immune system? Why? What MindBody intervention might be best?

Case 2

Your patient has rheumatoid arthritis. Do you want to strengthen, redirect, or weaken her immune system? Why? What MindBody interventions might be best?

Case 3

Your patient has asthma. Do you want to strengthen, redirect, or weaken his immune system? Why? What MindBody interventions might be best?

Case 4

Your patient reports "intense stress" many times in her day. What physical system is likely involved? What is your goal in approaching that system? What intervention would be helpful?

Case 5

Your patient experiences occasional tachycardia. Although under the care of a cardiologist, both she and your patient are interested in applying MindBody approaches. What area of the CNS is likely involved? What might you do to help by focusing a MindBody intervention on this area? What is a reasonable intervention?

Case 6

From a review of Chapter 1 and this chapter, what interventions are most likely to affect each body system? Speculate on how this might happen?

7

Three Essential Questions to Answer in Applying MindBody Interventions

Thus far, we have shared some current thoughts on just what interventions are used in MindBody medicine (Chapter 1). We then gave you some background on the areas that are influenced by these interventions: mental activities (Chapter 2) and the psychosocial phenomena (Chapter 4) associated with these mental activities. In Chapter 7, we help you better understand how to apply MindBody interventions to strengthen or change these mental activities and psychosocial phenomena to improve health.

A patient with skin rash and temperomandibular joint (TMJ) difficulties presents for help in employing MindBody interventions. To help her best, we must answer three questions:

1. Do we focus first on the presenting problem, applying MindBody techniques directly to the problem (e.g., hypnosis with imagery)? Note that in this text we refer to this approach of directly focusing on the presenting problem as the *direct* approach.
2. Do we focus first on the psychosocial phenomena contributing to the presenting problem (i.e., finding possible underlying issues such as stress, tension, and lack of support that may be contributing to her condition and addressing those issues first)? Note that in the text we refer to this approach of focusing on the contributing psychosocial phenomena first as the *indirect* approach.
3. Regardless of the direct or indirect approach, what will be the best MindBody intervention for her at this time?

This chapter will help you to assess which avenue of approach to take (direct or indirect) and to assess what might be the most powerful intervention. These are challenging questions to answer. Many patients, physicians, and other practicing health care professionals believe that the direct approach is always correct (e.g., help the person suffering with TMJ difficulties using medication, hypnosis, imagery or meditation, or whatever as long as you tackle the problem head on). Unfortunately, healing is not always so simple. Many physical problems are associated with psychosocial issues (remember Chapter 4) that need to be addressed first (the indirect approach) (e.g., stress, tension, lack of social support, negative self-talk, anger, etc. usually need addressing before the overt presenting problem is addressed). If these underlying issues are not addressed first, then addressing the presenting problem with a MindBody intervention is not likely to produce much success. If you do not help the patients manage their stress, then it will be more challenging to help them manage their suppressed immune system, which is associated with high stress.

A. GOALS

1. To have a deeper understanding of the direct and indirect approaches in applying MindBody interventions.
2. To learn questions to ask to obtain a clearer understanding regarding what intervention focus to take (direct or indirect).
3. To learn what type of information is useful in deciding on a particular intervention for a given patient situation.

B. LEARNING OBJECTIVES

After working through this chapter, you will be able to

1. Ask accurate questions that focus on clarifying which intervention focus to take.
2. Accurately focus on the important information to apply the best intervention to a patient situation.

C. INFORMATION GUIDE

Let us consider the patient who experienced skin rash and TMJ difficulties. She had great stress from her relationship with her in-laws and from school obligations, she felt unsupported by her husband, and she was unable to express her emotions. All these psychosocial issues had to be addressed before using a direct assault on her problem. After 3 weeks of successful marital therapy (a MindBody intervention that is a type of psychotherapy), her rash had gone away. She felt in control and stress free and had dealt with the issues of in-laws. At this time, we used hypnosis and imagery to approach her TMJ problem directly. The TMJ resolved after two sessions, and the lady has been symptom free for a year. (Remember the guidelines we put forth in the Introduction and Preface. This illustration of a patient's TMJ difficulties makes no scientific claims of cause and effect; we had no control group or true experimental design. However, we deliberately and methodically applied strategies that have good evidence of effectiveness in her type of situation, and the desired outcome was achieved.)

Which guidelines can you employ to assess the initial level of intervention needed (direct or indirect)? Which guidelines help decide the particular intervention to use (in this case, the use of hypnosis and imagery instead of another of the many MindBody interventions, e.g., art or biofeedback)?

This chapter will help you answer these questions. You will learn whether to assault a problem directly or indirectly; you will learn what might be the best approach for a particular patient. Before going further in this chapter, it will be helpful to have in mind a case and to apply actively what you study here to it.

In this section, we share questions to help you assess whether to approach a problem directly or indirectly. Then, we focus on questions to help you decide on the most powerful intervention to apply.

1. Direct or Indirect Approach

There are three questions that should be addressed to know whether to approach a health problem directly or indirectly:

1. Does the patient have healthful support?
2. Is the patient experiencing distress?
3. Is there a perceived positive result from the patient keeping the problem?

Does the Patient Have Healthful Support? Positive social support is associated with good health and patient adherence. Helping the patient to acquire positive social support is basic to enhancing good health. Therefore, regardless of the presenting problem, you might need to focus on helping the patient achieve this support. Possible questions include the following:

What do the people most important in your life say about your condition?
What does your family say about your condition? (Remember, positive comments here likely indicate positive support.)
Do you have a support system on which you can rely? (A "Yes" here likely indicates sufficient social support.)

Illustration

You are working with a patient who is experiencing chronic back pain. Since you know that positive social support is correlated with health (Chapter 4), you will want to understand this patient's perceptions and beliefs about his/her support system. (You also need to reach an understanding regarding whether the support system is truly supportive.) You also know from Chapter 4 that people with social support comply more with their treatment, and that a lack of social support could result in distress, which is associated with increased pain. Therefore, the first step before directly approaching the back pain is to help the patient get some sense of having social support. This is achieved by asking the three questions in the preceding paragraph. If these questions are not indicative of perceived and real social support, then your mission will be to assist the patient in acquiring social support (indirect approach) before employing measures to alleviate the back pain with a direct approach such as hypnosis or biofeedback (often, you may be surprised how the pain goes away or ceases to be important once the support is in place).

Is the Patient in Distress? As you learned from Chapter 4, distress can be a factor in many problems (e.g., increased bone fragility in women, vulnerability to the common cold, increased risk of cardiovascular problems); therefore, it is important to assist your patient in managing or eliminating distress prior to focusing directly on a presenting problem. Recall the patient with TMJ problems. The TMJ difficulty was first approached indirectly by helping her with her stressful family situation, and then the difficulty was directly addressed with hypnosis and imagery.

Here are questions to assist you in understanding a patient's level of stress:

Are there situations in your life that you feel are highly stressful?
If yes is your answer, what are they?
How do you manage these situations? (This answer will guide you regarding the effectiveness of the patient's attempted solutions, if any.)
Are you or have you in the past 2 years experienced any of the following: death of a loved one, divorce, loss of a job, major change in your life? (These areas are commonly stressful to most people in the American culture.) If so, tell me about it. (This sharing on the patient's part gives you insight regarding the effectiveness of your patient's management of stress.)

Illustration

The patient with TMJ problems and skin rash again provides a good illustration. In the assessment interview (asking questions regarding the patient's distress listed above), it was concluded that she was experiencing extreme distress (e.g., she perceived and believed herself trapped by school, in-laws, and marriage). We have good evidence that with this stress she is likely to have a suppressed immune system (this might relate to the skin rash), and possibly other conditions could be occurring of which she is unaware (e.g., increased bone fragility). Also, stress serves as a distraction that often interferes with treatment. Knowing this information, it was decided to help her manage her stress (indirect approach) prior to the hypnosis directed at the TMJ problems (direct approach).

Does the Patient Perceive Positive Results From Maintaining the Problem?
You need to discover if there are payoffs to the presenting problem that might interfere with approaching it directly. We have worked with many patients who in some way received a positive payoff for their illness. The following are examples:

- The experience of pain was perceived and believed to be a way of religious witnessing.
- A migraine resulted in the sufferer receiving special treats from members of the family.
- A child's asthma attack occurred every time his father began to beat his mother; the father stopped to take care of his son.
- A patient's painfulness when walking resulted in having a special chair made to give her comfort.
- A patient stated that he would like to feel well enough to return to work. When questioned, he shared that he was really afraid to return to work because when he was at work before his wife left him.
- A patient was told by a physician the patient respected that a rash would never go away. (The rash became a symbol of the physician's power, and for the patient, it was more secure to maintain the belief in the physician's power than for the rash to dissipate.)
- A patient's stomach pain resulted in stopping sexual intimacy whenever she wished to avoid a stressful family situation.

Illustration

A ten-year-old boy expresses headaches and wants to stay away from school every time there is a math test. The boy's headache results in a positive experience for him in the avoidance of school. Therefore, an indirect approach should be employed to eliminate the positive experience before we use a direct approach to eliminate the headache.

2. *Important Information Needed in Choosing the Best Intervention to Help a Patient's Situation*

1. You need to develop an understanding of the pathophysiology of the patient's disease. Therefore, review information on the pathophysiology of the disease/condition to be addressed. This information will assist you in making the intervention physiologically

correct (i.e., if the condition you are treating is one primarily involved in the hormone system, then you will build your intervention to address that system as part of the entire approach).

Illustration

Your patient has high blood pressure, and his laboratory values indicate that he is at risk for a heart attack. You will review the pathophysiology of his situation (by consulting with his physician, reading about the condition, or both). Through reviewing the pathophysiology, you better understand the physical factors. Therefore, you will understand that the stress hormone adrenaline is overly increased by the endocrine system when he is under stress. You will understand that adrenaline is likely implicated in raising blood pressure and increasing blood clotting time. All these phenomena are associated with high blood pressure and an increased risk of heart attack.

2. You need to review the interventions that are likely to work with the particular condition.
   Here you need to remember that understanding and successfully treating a condition using MindBody medicine requires knowledge of which interventions seem to help the condition directly and which psychosocial phenomena are related to that condition. Remember, these psychosocial phenomena may often need to be addressed prior to or along with your direct focus on the physical condition.

Illustration

You review Chapter 1 and Appendix B for interventions that seem to help the patient with the high blood pressure and heart attack risk directly (recall that examples of which intervention best influences which condition are found in both Chapter 1 and Appendix B). You learn from this review that meditation, psychotherapy, Hatha yoga, biofeedback, and music therapy have been shown to control blood pressure.

You might also review Chapter 4 for a reminder of which psychosocial phenomena may relate to the condition. You know from Chapter 4 that his condition may be associated with certain psychosocial factors: uncontrolled anger, anxiety, depression, unforgiving attitude, hopelessness, or stress. After talking with the patient, you discover that he is under a high amount of stress. In your review, you are reminded that stress is controlled by meditation, psychotherapy, expressive writing, humor, and hypnosis.

Now, you are aware of both direct and indirect interventions for his condition. Conveniently, with this particular condition you might utilize the same intervention (e.g., meditation). However, armed with the understanding of the pathophysiology of his condition, your approach can be more sophisticated than simply offering stress management. You could also focus on the hormone system itself (Chapter 6) and perhaps help the patient change the adrenaline flow (e.g., imagery of the hormone adrenaline being minimized and returning back to normal). Remember this is more speculative at this time.

3. You need to understand the patient's openness/readiness for an appropriate intervention.
   Therefore you need to understand the following:
   a. The patient's interest and knowledge: What interventions are they interested in using (e.g., is the patient interested in visual imagery as a way of improving their immune system?)?
   b. The patient's belief and perception about his or her condition and the possible intervention: What does the patient perceive and believe will truly help the situation (e.g., does the patient believe that meditation would truly help reduce stress?)?
   c. The patient's experience with the intervention: What has the patient or someone significant to them used with success (e.g., patient's close relative used visual imagery and believed it enhanced her stress control)?
   d. The patient's external limitations, such as time/money: What can be done effectively in a short time (e.g., the patient feels using humor and laughter could be done with limited time investment and help his high blood pressure)?

SUGGESTED READING

Astin, J., et al. (2003). Mind-Body medicine. State of the science, implication for practice. *Journal of the American Board of Family Practice, 16,* 131–147.

Galper, D.I., Taylor, A.G., & Cox, D.J. (2003). Current status of mind-body intervention for vascular complication of diabetes. *Family Community Health, 26,* 34–40. [This is good update on a MindBody intervention for a physical condition. It also gives guidance in assessing the usefulness of MindBody interventions.]

Marcus, J., Elkins, G., & Mott, F. (2003). The integration of hypnosis into a model of palliative care. *Integrative Cancer Therapy, 2,* 365–370.

Martelli, M.F., et al. (2004). Psychological, neurological and medical consultation, assessment and management of pain. *Journal of Head Trauma Rehabilitation, 19,* 10–18. [The authors give us insight and guidelines in accurate assessment for application of MindBody medicine.]

Pelletier, K.R. (2004). Mind-body medicine in ambulatory care. An evidence-based assessment. *Journal of Ambulatory Care Management, 27,* 25–42. [This article is useful for reviewing important factors in assessment.]

D. EXERCISES

Analyze and apply the information learned in this chapter to the following client situations:

Client Situation 1

A 42-year-old female patient presents complaining of chronic back pain and difficulty sleeping. She has been married 15 years and has two children; a girl 10 and a boy 12. She reports a "lack of connection" with her husband and difficulty communicating with her son. As she talks to you, you discern a somewhat hopeless attitude and lack of a sense of strength on her part. She tells you that she wishes she could have less back pain and sleep more.

Practice applying the questions from this chapter to learn if you should approach her pain and insomnia directly or first manage issues that may be affecting the pain and insomnia (the indirect approach). Then, discover information to help you decide which intervention would be best.

Application of Information from Chapter 7

Do you focus on her back pain and insomnia directly, or do you address underlying issues of stress and support (indirect approach)?

Does she have helpful support?

She reports a "lack of connection" and difficulty communicating with her son. Does this indicate low support? Also, does she have the support of friends? Does she belong to clubs, church groups, or other support services outside the family? If you determine that she needs positive social support, then this is important to include in your treatment plan before addressing or at least while addressing the back pain and insomnia.

Is she experiencing distress?

Does her present life situation and somewhat hopeless attitude indicate a feeling of being trapped and lack of hope (i.e. distress)? If so, then you will need to assist her to manage this.

Is there a perceived positive result from having pain and insomnia?

Is it the only way to get something for herself (e.g., attention, excuse not to do something, etc.)? If it is, then you will need to help her meet these needs in a more healthful manner. After you assist the client to take care of these issues (indirect approach), you may be surprised how the pain becomes less of an issue, and sleep returns. However, if this is not the case to her satisfaction, then you will need to apply interventions directly focused on modifying the pain and insomnia.

The following important information is needed to choose the best intervention for this patient:

Review information on the pathophysiology of both chronic back pain and insomnia. Which physical systems might be involved in her pain and insomnia? For example, if it is evident that the central nervous system is important in this situation, then focus on that system as part of your treatment.

Review interventions that seem to help these conditions. There is evidence that some interventions will address insomnia directly (e.g., meditation, psychotherapy, and humor/laughter). However, insomnia is often related to anxiety, depression, or stress. If her insomnia is related to one of these, then you can chose from several MindBody interventions that address the particular need (e.g., meditation lowers stress and anxiety, cognitive-behavioral therapy helps decrease anxiety and depression, expressive writing will help with stress and depression). Many interventions assist in pain management (e.g., imagery, meditation, psychotherapy, hypnosis, music therapy, energy focus).

Finally, you would answer Questions 3a–d to help make whatever intervention you may chose appropriate to this particular patient.

Client Situation 2

A 22-year-old male client arrives at the dental office with a terrible toothache. He reports that he has not experienced a toothache for a long time. X-rays show a root canal infection, indicating that the tooth had to come out. The client indicates that he is very anxious about this procedure. The dentist recommends a direct intervention using imagery or self-hypnosis to calm the patient during the time of the local anesthesia.

Was the dentist correct to recommend a direct intervention, or should he have recommended an indirect intervention? What would you recommend? What other type of direct intervention might be appropriate (refer to Chapter 1)?

8

Applying What You Have Learned to Patient Care

If you have read, studied, and worked through these chapters to this point, you have covered much information. This information is basic, but it is the foundation you can use to develop deeper understanding and skills in MindBody medicine. Even with this basic material, you have learned to think in a way to help you on your road to using MindBody medicine. In this chapter, we guide you in bringing what you have learned together and applying it to real cases. We do this by sharing the significant questions to be answered and illustrate for you the application of the answers to develop a treatment plan. The questions to be answered are presented in the Information Guide. We then take you through the answers and help you bring it together with a tentative treatment plan. We include other scenarios in the Exercise section for you to apply your knowledge. You will need to review the previous chapters to do this application well. This review will reinforce the information you have learned.

A. GOAL

This chapter's goal is to be able to apply information learned to patient situations.

B. LEARNING OBJECTIVES

After working through this chapter, you will be able to

1. Secure information to answer important MindBody questions.
2. Use information from these answers to assist a patient.

C. INFORMATION GUIDE

This is a list of basic questions to help you apply MindBody medicine to a patient situation:

1. What mental activities are the patient using (Chapter 2)?
2. What psychosocial phenomena are significant in the patient's situation (Chapter 6)?
3. How can you decide whether to address the problem directly or indirectly (Chapter 7)?
4. What physical systems might be an important focus in this situation (Chapter 5)?
5. What interventions might work with the patient's health issues (Chapter 1)?
6. What might be the best intervention for this patient and the patient's situation (Chapter 6)?

Case 1

Ms. A is a 45-year-old female referred to you by her oncologist since Ms. A has been diagnosed with breast cancer. Her oncologist knows that total care for this patient requires helping her with her mental activities (e.g., the patient's perception of what is happening, her imagination, etc.). Ms. A is a little skeptical but wants to do all she can to be as well as possible. You notice in your interview with her that she is an intelligent, creative thinker but passive. She says up to now she was "well organized" but is "falling apart" after the diagnosis. She uses many limiting terms (e.g., "can't," "never," etc.), and these terms are part of her negative self-talk (e.g., "I guess I'll just die younger than I had thought"). You also learn that her job as a teacher carries high demands and expectations, but she perceives, believes, and tells herself that she has no power to change things.

Analysis of Case 1

In analyzing Case 1, we take each question listed in the Information Guide and discuss some possible insight that might apply to this case as well as reminders of possible intervention strategies. After this discussion, a more detailed presentation of what was done and is being done in work with Ms. A is presented. In this presentation, *italicized* words are used to help you focus on material that relates to questions 1 through 6 and answers that are given to these questions Therefore, when a mental activity, MindBody intervention, or psychosocial phenomenon is mentioned, it will appear in *italics*.

1. What mental activities is she employing (Chapter 2)?

   She is employing the following mental activities: *perception, belief, memory,* and *calculation.* She *perceives* and *believes* herself to be limited (e.g., she employs limiting terms such as "can't" and "never," and she *perceives* and *believes* she has no power to change things at her job). Using her *imagination* and *memory,* she states that she will "just die younger than I had thought." It is likely that she is *imagining* scenarios around her illness and fate, *calculating* outcomes, and using her *memory* of other people and events that she *believes* relate to her. As you work with her, you will want to change the illness-enhancing content in these mental activities. Since she *perceives* and *believes* herself to be limited and has *memories* that tend to be focused on bad outcomes, you might include in your interventions ways to change these *perceptions* and *beliefs* and reinterpret/reframe the *memories* into a more powerful sense of hope and possibility. For example, you could employ simple education regarding her *perceptions* and *self-imagery* to focus on different healthful *perceptions* and use *cognitive-behavioral therapy* to change her *perceptions, beliefs,* and *calculations* about her situation.

2. What are the psychosocial phenomena related to her condition that might be important in her treatment (Chapter 4)?

   Social support: There is good evidence that people with cancer live longer when they perceive, believe, and objectively have positive social support.

   Fighting spirit: The attitude that "I can live life well and even delay or overcome this" may contribute to her living longer.

   Optimism: This quality is associated with longevity.

   High stress: This is associated with suppressed immunity, which could be detrimental to fighting cancer.

   Depression: Depression is associated with lowered immunity.

   Any or all of these may have to be addressed in treating Ms. A.

3. How can you decide to address the problem directly or indirectly (Chapter 7)?

   Initially, you will want to address the problem indirectly if basic psychosocial phenomena relate to her situation need changing. You can focus on the following areas to help you decide:

   You will want to know about her current support system. Does she *perceive, believe,* and in your clinical judgment have true social support? In her case, you would want her to have several loving friends or family members who would listen to her, do things with her, be optimistic, focus on the here-and-now quality of life, and avoid overemphasis on her condition.

   You will want to know about her distress. You know that the diagnosis itself is stressful. Additional indications of distress are her *perception* and *belief* that she is "falling apart," her use of many limiting terms (e.g., "can't"), and her *perception* and *belief* that she has high demands on her but little power. Therefore, indirectly you need to help her find positive social support and manage distress first to help her with her cancer.

In addition, review the psychosocial phenomena listed under the answers to Question 2 and help her correct or enhance these as appropriate.

4. What physical systems are important in this situation (Chapter 6)?

You will need to confer with her oncologist to understand the physical systems involved in her situation. The immune system will be the key. Also, understanding the location and pathophysiology of the cancer and the discomfort she may experience from both it and her treatment will be important. This information will help you focus your interventions more accurately on the appropriate system both anatomically and physiologically.

5. What interventions might work with her health issues (Chapter 1 and Appendix B)?

In reviewing your knowledge from Chapter 1, you can develop an idea of what interventions have been demonstrated to help a person in Ms. A's situation. Keep in mind that it will not be until you answer Question 6 that you will know which of these interventions are possibly best suited for her specific case. Knowing the diagnosis and possible biochemical/physical treatments she might have to endure, you might consider the following interventions (remember, in some illness situations the actual medical interventions may cause difficulties such as pain, anxiety, etc.; helping with these experiences may need to be part of your approach):

Meditation: Lowers stress and anxiety in cancer patients and helps with sleep problems.

Imagery: Employed successfully by some patients to shrink tumors.

Group therapy: Improves mood and seems to extend life span in patients with breast cancer.

Psychotherapy: Helps with any depression or anxiety, managing invasive medical procedures more comfortably, modifying pain, and correcting insomnia.

Hypnosis: Helps to enhance the immune system, correct sleep problems, manage pain, and assist in more comfortably undergoing medical procedures.

Music therapy: helps reduce pain, increase immunity, and lower anxiety and assists in preparation for medical procedures.

Yoga: Useful aid to relieve pain.

Positive self-talk: Helps eliminate the sensation of pain and improve a sense of well-being.

Energy focus: Decreases or eliminates sensation of pain.

Humor and laughter: Combats insomnia, lowers pain perception, and enhances the immune system.

Expressive writing: Helps relieve stress and depression.

6. What might be the best intervention for this patient (Chapter 7)?

From the interventions that might help in her condition (listed for Question 5), discover which may be the best for her particular situation. Answers to the following will help you make this discovery:

What do significant people in her life say about the different interventions, especially her oncologist? Like any intervention, it is helpful for Ms. A to *perceive* and *believe* the intervention will help. This *perception* and *belief* is strengthened by positive input from people she respects and trusts.

Has she tried any of these interventions before? Was she successful? Does she feel it helped? Remember she is a "little skeptical" and "creative." Make sure she is comfortable with any intervention in that it makes sense to her intelligence. Employ her creativity.

Discussion of Actual Interventions

This process could be applied to any case.

When you meet Ms. A for the first time and throughout your work in MindBody medicine, you are expected to be able to apply basic skills from interviewing/*psychotherapy* training. (These skills, such as empathy, refocusing, reconnecting, reframing, reinforcing, etc., are presumed to be in the basic competence of a professional employing MindBody medicine before the person is in a position to offer assistance in its application.)

Therefore, in the initial interview you will build rapport and obtain basic information. In doing this, you will want to understand Ms. A's goals, what she is interested in doing, her family's and significant other's role in her health, and a complete picture of the psychosocial phenomena that might affect her life. As you gather this information, you will listen for her use of limiting terms such as "can't," "never," and "should" as these will give you insight regarding her openness to accepting that she can change. Be aware of what mental activities she employs. You also need to know what she has tried in MindBody medicine and her opinion of the intervention's usefulness. Throughout this process, be aware of the need to help her have hope. Finally, remember the importance of consulting with the treating physician, thus garnering better insight into the nature of the illness, its location, and its pathophysiology (this will help you in reviewing the physical systems most important to this illness; in Ms. A's case, it will likely be the immune system).

In interviewing Ms. A, the content of the principal mental activities she was employing (*perceptions, beliefs, memories,* and *calculations*) concerning her situation should become evident. In this case, Ms. A's use of mental activities were valuable help. She had a *perception* that her employment of MindBody medicine could be helpful in some way. She expressed a *belief* in the possibility of MindBody interventions. This was helped by her *memories* of how she experienced MindBody connection in the past (e.g., turning red when embarrassed). Finally, she could *calculate* that she had a good chance at enhanced quality of life through her use of MindBody medicine.

Because of these qualities, Ms. A was very open and interested in MindBody approaches. The decision was made to approach her situation both directly and indirectly. Remember to remain aware of her mental activities, such as *perception,* and how their content may or may not be changing. This is the foundation of MindBody medicine for this is the mind at work. So, if Ms. A continued to *perceive* that she had no hope, it is imperative that she be helped to change this perception. These changes in mental activity usually occur during intervention with appropriate MindBody techniques. If the destructive content of a mental activity continues, then that destructive content is often handled directly by *cognitive therapy, imagery,* or *hypnosis.* Ms. A responded well to *cognitive therapy* and *hypnosis* in this regard. This change could also be assisted by educating her regarding what MindBody interventions might be helpful in her situation by explaining some of the research and the dynamics of the interventions with examples.

It is important to investigate the psychosocial phenomena that affect her life and focus on helping her to be in as healthy a place as possible concerning these (indirect approach). You would examine her *social support* and guide her to encourage *positive social support* situations, which for her were her family and her church group. Also, explain the importance of the *fighting spirit, optimism,* and avoiding *high stress* and *depression.*

Ms. A was taught *positive self-talk* to help her develop a *fighting spirit.* This was strengthened through *imagery* and *role-play.* To help develop *optimism, humor* was employed. She should be helped to practice seeing the positive in situations. To help her combat the *high stress,* consider these three areas: changing the situations of stress; avoiding the situations of stress; and reinterpreting the situations perceived as stressful.

1. School might be made less stressful by teaching Ms. A assertiveness and helping her approach her principal to have her work modified (her shyness in this area was helped by the use of *hypnosis*).
2. Review situations to avoid and practice how to avoid them (helping her to have a plan of behavior).
3. Employ *cognitive-behavioral therapy* to stop her negative self-talk about both work and her condition.
4. Stress in general could be lowered by developing with her a program of *meditation,* exercise, and *biofeedback.*
5. Finally, the *depression* would be addressed by *psychotherapy* and *meditation.*

As you should recall, many of these initial interventions are indirect. They address those psychosocial phenomena that are associated with her cancer. Examples of direct interventions to employ are *visual imagery* under deep *hypnotic trance* (here, focus on the pathophysiology of the cancer, employing Ms. A's image of her white cells accurately attacking the tumor and cutting off its blood supply); *prayer* (consistent with Ms. A's belief system); and *energy focus*. She should also be enrolled in a *group therapy* program.

D. EXERCISES

Apply the guidelines learned in this chapter to these two cases. You may want to refer to earlier chapters for help with the answers. Check your answers against ours.

Case 2

You have been requested to consult regarding a 35-year-old male patient with hypertension. The patient and the patient's physician are open to MindBody medicine, and they are interested in information you may share from this area that might help the patient. When you interview the patient, you find him cooperative. These are some facts that he shares about his life and condition: He tells you how his job is interesting but challenging; in fact, he must often react aggressively to get the job accomplished (he is a foreman at the local refinery). He admits that there are times when he loses his temper. He has a strong belief that "if you do something, do it right." Many workers, he perceives, do not care. He has identified some of their work as totally unacceptable and believes and feels that he is responsible for "making it right." He feels that he has a lot of responsibility but not many options because of the workers' union. He also reports some anxiety and at times feeling a "little down." He says he is open to try anything; he has a good imagination and has long been interested in Eastern religion.

1. What mental activities does he use the most?
2. What are the psychosocial phenomena related to his condition that might be important in his treatment?
3. How can you decide to address the problem directly or indirectly?
4. What physical systems are important in this situation?
5. What interventions might work for his condition?
6. What might be the best intervention for this patient and why?

The following are our answers to Case 2.

1. What mental activities is he using?

   He seems to be using *perception* and *belief.* These mental activities are likely influenced by his *memory* of events and things he has learned. He *believes* that he must act aggressively, that "if you do something, do it right"; that many workers do not care; that he "must make work go right"; and that he has few options. You will need to discover if his *perception* and *belief* about his workers and responsibility relate to his hypertension. To discover this, consider these questions:

   a. Does his *belief* that he must act aggressively add to his stress?
   b. Is his *perception* of his worker's attitudes interpreted correctly, or does he need help in seeing their attitude and behavior in a positive light?
   c. Are his *perception* and *belief* that he is the one to "make work right" correct?
   d. What are his early *memories* about life messages about himself, his responsibilities, and work, and do they need modifying before he will be open to change?

   He says his job is "interesting and challenging" but feels he must take control at times. In any case, if he *perceives* and *believes* what he does is a challenge in which he has some control and dedication, then he is in a healthier situation than if he saw it otherwise.

   He mentions his anger. You know from Chapter 4 that managing anger and exercising forgiveness are associated with lowering blood pressure in hypertensive individuals, so helping with his anger is important. Checking to see if he holds anger and the like because of his perception and belief that some workers are unreliable and he has to do it for them are part of his perception.

   Insofar as these issues are part of his hypertension, then our interventions would be focused on possibly changing the way he *perceives* and what he believes about his work environment and responsibility.

2. What are the psychosocial phenomena related to his condition that might be important in his treatment?

   In reviewing Chapter 4, you are reminded that, with hypertension, optimism, constructive management of anger, and forgiving perceived wrongs are all associated with lowering blood pressure. Also, stress, unmanaged anger, and depression are associated with hypertension. The short description in Case 2 gives you several clues regarding the possibility of anger, stress, and perhaps depression: He admits to losing his temper; feeling like he must do the job himself to get it done correctly because "some of their work is totally unacceptable"; feeling like he has "lots of responsibility but few options" (a possible source of stress and even depression); and tells you he has been feeling a "little down." We would review the issues with the patient and consider helping him correct these needs in our treatment approach.

3. How do you decide to address the problem directly or indirectly?

Understanding the general psychosocial phenomena that relate to the patient and the patient's specific problem helps you make this decision. You should always screen for stress and social support. As you recall from Chapter 4, distress and the lack of social support are associated with many health problems, including hypertension. You should address these before (indirect approach) or along with directly intervening with the problem. In addition to distress and social support, you would review other psychosocial phenomena that relate to health and if any of these are interfering with the patient's well-being, then address them first or along with the direct interventions.

In working with our foreman from Case 2, we decided that there are psychosocial phenomena that likely influence his hypertension. We elected to help him with his stress, anger, and mood before directly approaching the hypertension. In the situations that could not be changed, such as the limits imposed by the workers' union, we focused on helping the patient modify his *perceptions* and *beliefs* about what was needed along with learning to deal with issues with calm assertiveness rather than aggressiveness. Our techniques are shared in the answers to Question 6.

We would also check on his *perception* and *belief* about his support system. Positive social support is an important factor in helping with stress (stress relates to hypertension), and we would help in securing positive social support if he does not have it.

4. What physical systems are involved?

Of course, all three physical systems are involved in the healing process. In helping with his stress, temper, and mood, we are conscious of the role played by the central nervous system in the form of *belief* and self-talk. In looking at hypertension directly, we are aware of the autonomic nervous system. The "so what?" here is to be aware of these systems and focus our interventions as much as possible in modifying anything about the system that would help. We addressed the central nervous system by changing his limiting self-talk ("shoulds" and "oughts") about his perceptions and beliefs concerning his limitations. To address the autonomic system and directly focus on hypertension, we would employ interventions to enhance his parasympathetic system (i.e., help him relax).

5. What interventions generally work for his condition?

In helping with stress, temper, mood, and strong beliefs about always "doing it right," the following are often effective: meditation, cognitive-behavioral psychotherapy, hypnosis with imagery, support groups, expressive writing, and poetry writing. In addressing the hypertension directly, energy focus, art, psychotherapy, meditation, and hypnosis have been used successfully.

6. What intervention might be the best for this particular patient?
   We know that he is open, interested in Eastern religion, and takes responsibility. Our approach was to help him as follows:
   - Modify his perceptions and beliefs by using *cognitive-behavioral therapy.* This involved having him address some early memories of how he should behave and correcting his general beliefs that he "has to do it all."
   - We helped him change some of his limiting terms and perception of "few options" with cognitive therapy.
   - We also began assisting him to learn meditation (his interest in Eastern religion helped here) and employing this skill to help him lower stress and anxiety and control anger.
   - Finally, we addressed his hypertension directly by cognitive-behavioral therapy and hypnosis with imagery that he chose and directed (remembering he likes to take responsibility).

Critically review our approach, compare it with your thoughts, and review the relevant chapter. This will assist you in increasing your skills in applying the material.

9

MindBody Medicine for Today's Health Care Consumer

In Chapter 9, we present areas we have found from our practice to be relevant to today's health care consumer, which at one time or another will be all of us. It is important as a health care consumer to keep in mind the integration of mind and body. The more we understand human behavior and cognition, the more we appreciate the truth of this interconnection. Even though many works on this subject seem to separate the mind from the body, we attempt to avoid this separation and hope the use of the term *MindBody* helps emphasize that goal. Of course, in this book we focus on this integration as it might apply to health and the prevention and curing of illness. In this chapter, we present a short discussion of thoughts of wellness rather than illness. All of this is part of a reemphasis on the importance of a holistic approach.

A. GOALS

1. To better understand the interconnection of mind and body in health.
2. To better understand how MindBody medicine may be involved in developing wellness and health.
3. To review thoughts on the holistic approach to health.

B. LEARNING OBJECTIVES

After working through this chapter, you will be able to

1. List at least three MindBody medicine interventions that may be employed to enrich health rather than just "cure" an illness.
2. List characteristics of health.
3. Apply two MindBody techniques to a client situation to assist in the development of health.

C. INFORMATION GUIDE

You are aware by now in your study of MindBody medicine and MindBody interventions of how integrated the mind and body are. In this section, we share a short reminder of this integration in illness, and then we change our focus to considerations of applying MindBody intervention in the development of health.

The Integration of Mind and Body

There is evidence that indicates that as many as half of all patients who visit physicians have physical symptoms that are directly caused by emotions; other researchers report the figure to be as high as 90% (Hafen, Karren, Frandsen, & Smith, 1996).

As you should recall from Chapter 4, conditions that are usually considered physical, such as cancer, pain, and even diabetes, are often associated with psychological factors such as stress. In reviewing Chapter 4, you are reminded of how stress can leave the immune system vulnerable to physical disease, increase the vulnerability to cardiovascular disease, and even increase blood sugar in diabetes. In addition, a person who receives the diagnosis of a severe physical disease often experiences enormous psychological stress, and that kind of stress can in turn influence the immune system (Achterberg, Dossey, & Kolkmeier, 1994).

To help clarify this integration of the mind and body and the role of MindBody intervention, consider the following example: According to some researchers, as many as 70% of all people who go to a gastrointestinal specialist have irritable bowel syndrome, a mixture of pain, diarrhea, constipation, nausea, and sometimes vomiting. One fourth of these gastroenterology patients have major depression. After receiving MindBody intervention for these symptoms, 89% of the patients reported less pain as a result; 96% had less diarrhea, 90% had less constipation, 92% were less nauseated, and 81% had less vomiting. Researchers who conducted the study concluded that the symptoms of irritable bowel syndrome were seen as a physical expression of emotions caused by recent loss or ongoing stressful life situations. This is a reminder of how MindBody interventions are helpful in treating illness (Hafen et al., 1996).

Application of MindBody Medicine in Wellness Rather Than Illness

As with many traditional Western medical interventions, MindBody medicine research and practice have been largely focused on interventions in the illness process. Usually, these interventions are in the form of ameliorating conditions associated with a disease process, such as nausea with chemotherapy, stress, and the like. There are also some reports of attempting to apply MindBody interventions to the actual curing of illness (the references to these are abundant in both Chapter 1 and Appendix B).

Several trends today invite us to expand that focus not only to the amelioration of illness conditions or the curing of illness, but also to the actual prevention of illness and the enhancement of health (e.g., the Harvard Medical School program in MindBody medicine; Allison, 1999; Chamberlin, 2006; National Institutes of Health, 1994; Richman et al., 2005; Seligman et al., 2005). With this in mind, we thought it would be valuable to give some consideration to just what might be the qualities of good health and emotional well-being and how MindBody medicine could be involved in promoting these qualities.

Health, like love and happiness, is a challenge to define. Often, *health* is defined and discussed in the negative: what is lack of health rather than what is good health. That is, health is considered from the point of view of lack of illness, discomfort, or distress (U.S. Public Health Service and World Health Organization). As practitioners of MindBody medicine, we suggest that you consider health and emotional well-being from the vantage point of the positive, what they are rather than what they are not. We share definitions that we hope will assist in better understanding this positive focus.

Wellness: The process of living at one's highest possible level as a whole person and promoting the same for others. The ability to use positive lifestyle habits to enjoy health.

Health: A condition in which a system functions in a manner needed to maintain its ability to grow, reproduce, and interact in a way that enables the system to enhance the society in which the system lives. In a human, this is translated as follows: A person is able to comfortably do those activities needed so that the person is able to grow, reproduce, and interact with other humans and the environment in ways that are helpful for both the individual and the others. Let us take this somewhat abstract description and make it more useful by answering the question, "What are the signs and symptoms of this healthy person?" with more concrete descriptors. This is better understood by focusing on the physical, emotional, and social aspects of a person.

Physically: A person is healthy when

- All body systems function in such a manner to allow the person to achieve continued growth, reproduction, and physical interactions appropriate to age. Such things as appropriate cell reproduction, heart and lung function, and muscle growth activity would indicate this.

Emotionally: A person is healthy when able to

- Approach each experience as an opportunity for being creative, happy, helpful.
- Take responsibility for personal success.

- Take responsibility for personal shortcomings.
- Be able to feel love for self and others.

Socially: A person is healthy when able to

- Interact with others in a manner that promotes the others' well-being as well as their own. Emotional and social health might include these characteristics reported in the current research on the area of wellness: kindness, fairness, authenticity, gratitude, and open-mindedness (Seligman et al., 2005).

Examples of Applying MindBody Medicine to Promote Wellness

In this section, we take each point listed and make some observations on applying MindBody techniques for enhancing a person's health and well-being. Any of the techniques presented in Chapter 1 might be applicable. Here, we present illustrations to help you better understand (if possible, we draw from our experience in using this approach). Like many of the interventions discussed throughout this book, there is little research in this area. So, we are working on that beginning stage of good science by reporting observations from our work with people, drawing from the principles inherent in the interventions, and proposing the hypothesis that there is some association, possibly even cause and effect. The exciting part is up to us and you to challenge this hypothesis by applying solid research to these areas.

Physical Health

Example 1

- *Goal:* To enhance a person (referred to here as *client* since the person is not in a patient role) to function at an optimum level while engaged in a sport activity.
- *Interventions employed*: Imagery, hypnosis.
- *Illustration of application:* The first author has worked with professional athletes to assist them in enhancing their physical health as well as success in their sport. A combination of visual imagery under hypnosis was the intervention utilized. The client would receive the suggestion of seeing himself play the sport in an ideal fashion, feel invigorated, and imagine his entire body system being in top performance. After applying this approach, clients have consistently reported achieving their goals.

Example 2

- *Goal:* To assist a client in the enhancement of her immune system.
- *Interventions employed:* Meditation, yoga.
- *Illustration of application:* A client requested help in strengthening her immune system. She was going to be working in a foreign area

where she would experience high stress and possible exposure to disease. She was familiar with imagery and self-hypnosis, which she had been employing. In addition, she felt that any other nonchemical approach might be useful. She was taught meditation and some basic yoga postures, breathing, and moves. Both these interventions helped with bringing her to a deep state of relaxation. This relaxation would help lower her stress and protect her immune system. In addition, you might recall (Chapter 1) that meditation seems to assist in strengthening the immune system.

Emotional Health

Example 1

- *Goal*: To help a client approach life as an opportunity for being creative, happy, helpful.
- *Intervention employed:* Psychotherapy, music therapy.
- *Illustration of application:* By undergoing 6 weeks of cognitive-behavioral therapy, a client increased her sense of well-being as she increased her awareness of her own options in life and her positive self-talk. The simple act of listening to enjoyable music on a regular basis helped her to review her perceptions and beliefs about her life as an opportunity for growth and achievement.

Example 2

- *Goal*: To help a client be open to accepting and giving love.
- *Intervention employed:* Yoga, support groups.
- *Example of application:* A client found that her involvement in yoga gave her a deeper sense of her own value, the importance of the MindBody connection, and the value of others (i.e., she is lovable and so are others). Involvement in a weekly support group was an eye-opener for one client when she got the clear message from fellow group members that she was likable.

Social Health

Example 1

- *Goal:* To interact with others in a manner that promotes the other's well-being as well as one's own well-being; that is, developing the characteristics of kindness, fairness, authenticity, gratitude, open-mindedness.
- *Interventions employed*: Meditation, humor/laughter.
- *Illustration of application*: The first author assisted a client in learning mindfulness meditation. One of the products of regular meditation (i.e., daily meditation for about 20 minutes each time) is an achievement of a deep sense of being calmly in the here and now. This practice enhances one's ability to let go of past and future concerns, be

more compassionate, and be more attuned to others. After 2 months of meditation, the client reported the ability to more calmly interact with others in a happy, helpful manner.

Example 2

- *Goal:* To assist a client in feeling more at ease in a social situation.
- *Interventions employed:* Humor and laughter.
- *Example of intervention:* The use of humor and laughter were interventions reported by a client who wished to be more at ease and attuned to others. She perceived and believed that the humor/laughter approach helped her to take her self less seriously, and hence she was less self-conscious around others and could be more attuned to their needs.

The Holistic Approach

MindBody medicine is integral to a holistic approach in that it encompasses the whole person. The following is a definition of the holistic approach: "An approach that includes physical symptoms, emotional states, social and physical conditions, the person in an environment, the cultural influences, and cognitive interpretations" (Cowles, 2004).

MindBody medicine is an important part of the holistic approach and must be included as such. To emphasize, MindBody medicine should be included in both the treatment of illness and the development of wellness and health because without making use of mental activities, healing cannot take place or wellness develop. If we are to solve human health problems with a good result, then this holistic approach in health care and health management is the answer.

As Andrew Weil has shared, the function of healing depends on the operation of all the systems, especially on the mental activities of our mind and other nonphysical components of our beings (Weil, 1997).

It is also known that people who use a holistic health care approach do so for the following reasons: to prevent disease recurrence and to improve quality of life during a chronic illness; out of dissatisfaction with the physician-patient relationship and a desire for a more patient-centered approach; and out of disenchantment with the current health care system ("Mind Body Medicine News," 2005).

SUGGESTED READING

Achterberg, J., Dossey, B., & Kolkmeier, L. (1994). *Rituals of Healing*. New York: Bantam Books. [We see this as a classic in helping the reader obtain a deeper insight into the use of MindBody interventions for developing health.]

Allison, N. (Ed.). (1999). *The Complete Body, Mind, and Spirit*. New York: Keats.

Chamberlin, J. (2006). A picture of health: A psychologist's multidimensional employee wellness initiative at the University of Missouri emphasizes mind-body health. *Monitor on Psychology, 57*, 30–31. [This short article presents an updated and interesting view of the possibilities of focusing on wellness in an established program.]

Cowles, C.A. (2004). *Social Work in the Health Field*. Binghamton, NY, Haworth Press.

Hafen, B.Q., Karren, K.J., Frandsen, K.J., & Smith, N.L. (1996). *Mind Body Health*. Needham Heights, MA: Simon & Schuster.

Mind-Body medicine news. (2005). *Advances, 21*, 33.

National Institutes of Health. (1993). New research frontiers in behavioral medicine. Washington, DC: U.S. Government Printing Office. [A useful "official" guide regarding the National Institutes of Health's conclusions concerning many MindBody interventions. The idea of health development and enhancement can be seen with some of the future research consideration.]

Richman, L., et al. (2005). Positive emotion and health: Going beyond the negative. *Health Psychology, 24*, 422–429. [This work invites the reader to consider the notion of a positive approach in health psychology.]

Seligman, M., et al. (2005). Positive psychology progress: Empirical validation of interventions. *American Psychologist, 60*, 410–421. [Dr. Seligman is a leading thinker in this area of applying psychology (hence MindBody medicine) to understanding, developing, and enriching the area of health promotion rather than just "curing" problems.]

Weil, A. (1997). *Eight Weeks to Optimum Health*. New York: Random House.

D. EXERCISES

These exercises will serve you best by applying them to real cases, preferably ones with which you may have worked. Their usefulness will be further increased by applying them to your life circumstances.

1. Just for a review, recall a time when you or someone you knew was ill. By reviewing this chapter (and others if needed), list how the mind played a role in the illness. You will be helped in this by reviewing the mental activities (Chapter 2).
2. Now, see if you can recall a situation when you or someone you knew employed MindBody medicine to feel better, such as using meditation to help reduce high blood pressure.
3. Change your focus from applying MindBody medicine to the curing of an illnesses to a focus on preventing an illness and enriching health. With this focus, review the three areas of health mentioned in this chapter: physical, emotional, and social. We shared examples of applying MindBody interventions to help prevent illness and enrich health by helping to enrich each area. In this exercise, we invite you to do the same. Practice applying a MindBody intervention to each area.
4. Review our thoughts on health and wellness. Critique them by adding dimensions or taking away the ones with which you do not

agree; justify your decision with references to publications or your own reasoning.

5. You are the master of your own voice: Make your own relaxation and imagery tapes. Imagery is discussed in our intervention chapter (Chapter 1). Write down your thoughts and record your voice. Use your name as you record exactly what you want to hear when you play your tape. Your voice is a powerful tool. You can even modulate your voice to increase the power of your words. Listen to your tapes several times a day or week. You could also play soft music that you find relaxing when you listen to your tape.
6. Reflect on the physical, emotional, and social areas of your life that could be made healthier. Set goals in each area. Apply MindBody interventions to achieve these goals. These ideas will be helpful:
   a. Make your own inventory: What are your strengths? How do you deal with old patterns of self-blame, worry, anger, self-pity, and any other patterns you may want to change in your life?
   b. Write out and analyze your old profile.
   c. Create a new wellness profile for yourself and stick to it.
   d. Chose one or two MindBody interventions from Chapter 1 to help you achieve your new goals (e.g., meditation to help you be more calm and focused; imagery to assist in envisioning yourself acting and feeling your goals).
   e. Measure your own success on a weekly basis by establishing a baseline; create a scale from 1 to 10 and record your success.
   f. Pursue your plan and celebrate your wellness and health with your family and friends.
7. Apply this chapter to the following cases:
   a. Describe Marcia's and Billy's life-school stressors and work with each using a health-and-wellness plan.

      Marcia is an energetic student at a local college. She is under pressure to compete with other students, and she thrives under pressure. Marcia seldom seems tired or discouraged to help people in the community. Marcia states that she does not need a wellness plan because she never seems to have enough time for herself, and she does not want to add additional tasks to her life.

      What is going on? What kind of MindBody intervention would you recommend for Marcia and provide your reasoning for it?
   b. Billy just started as a community college student and used to feel energetic most of the time. Now, he moves through his days more like a snail. Billy also turns down parties and prefers to spend time alone studying and developing new programs on his computer. He told his friend that he misses his family and friends back home.

      What kind of MindBody intervention would you recommend for Billy, and provide your reasoning for it?

10

Thoughts on the Future of MindBody Medicine

The interest in and popularity of MindBody medicine is rapidly growing. We see the evidence for this statement in the number of books and journal articles that cross our desks daily. Further evidence can be found in the number of books in bookstores in such areas as new age, self-enrichment, psychology, and so on. Although in our opinion many of these works tend to cover areas other than MindBody medicine (e.g., acupuncture, massage), they offer evidence of its popularity.

More important are the number of research projects we have come across in our reviews for this book. Again, it may be argued that many lack the best scientific approach (something we have found in the research literature on allopathic medicine as well), and many classified as MindBody are focused, like the popular press, on other than MindBody medicine. These publications demonstrate an interest in understanding the area of MindBody medicine.

In our opinion, MindBody medicine will be a major area of health care practice and research in the future. If you have studied the material in this book, then you have no doubt begun to think critically about the topic and, it is hoped, its place in the health care of the future. We hope that you have challenged our ideas, created some of your own, and given consideration to what MindBody medicine will be like in 20, 30, or 40 years. In this chapter, we place the Exercise section first. After you do the exercise, then read the Information Guide and compare your thoughts with those we have listed.

A. GOAL

The goal of the chapter is to develop a deeper understanding of how MindBody medicine might be in the future.

B. LEARNING OBJECTIVES

After working through this chapter, you will be able to

1. List areas that you believe will characterize MindBody medicine in the future.
2. List reasons to justify your belief.

C. EXERCISES

List your thoughts on the tools and procedures of MindBody medicine in the years to come. Before continuing, list those areas in which you think MindBody medicine might change. After you make these lists, we suggest you consider the areas we have listed. To further enrich this exercise, take time actually to write your answers to the questions. It will be interesting to discover in which areas your thoughts match our thoughts. You will find our thoughts on these areas developed in the Information Guide.

1. What types of testing might be employed in decision making in MindBody medicine?
2. What new MindBody interventions do you envision?
3. Do you believe any of the interventions mentioned in Chapter 1 will be shown to be of little or no use? If so, which?
4. Do you see a change in understanding mental activities and their uses?
5. Will energy play a more significant role in understanding and applying MindBody medicine? If yes, what and how?
6. What are your thoughts on the qualifications and training needed to apply the tools of MindBody medicine?

After making your list, then we invite you to compare your thoughts with ours in the Information Guide.

D. INFORMATION GUIDE

From our research in and teaching of MindBody medicine, we offer the following thoughts on its future:

1. Personality inventories that detect both state and trait features of personality will be refined or developed to help match personality characteristics with a particular MindBody intervention. For example, let us say a patient is given the Myers-Briggs-type indicator. Her personality preferences are shown from her answers to the indicator as introversion, intuition, thinking, and judging (i.e.,

being organized). Future research will focus on just what type of MindBody intervention might work for that particular constellation of personality preferences. This research will answer such questions as the following: Does an intuitive person respond better to cognitive therapy or expressive art when dealing with an illness? Does the introvert use biofeedback better than group support in their health needs?

2. There will be development of techniques or instruments to better clarify just how mental activity influences physical health and how physical health influences mental activity. These techniques/instruments will be designed to enhance our understanding of the association between the content of mental activities such as perception, belief, memory, imagination, and the like and a particular physical illness. They will better refine our knowledge regarding whether a mental activity really does influence physical health, how it might do that, and how physical health exactly influences mental activity. For example, these techniques/instruments might help us understand just what mechanism happens in such phenomena as shunting blood while under hypnosis. Thus, clarification will be given to such questions as how a person in trance, seemingly by just their perception and belief, can cause his or her blood to leave one part of the body and go to another.
3. Mental activity and MindBody interventions will be visualized by applying physical imaging instruments, for example, utilizing magnetic resonance imaging to visualize the brain activity when a patient *believes* that he or she will have great pain or employing a positron emission tomographic scan to visualize brain activity when using a MindBody intervention to change a belief.
4. There will be increased exposure to information in MindBody medicine. For example, there will be more formal course offerings in the schools of medicine, psychology, social work, graduate nursing, and the like. These will take the form of graduate seminars covering topic such as those presented in this book, and they will be offered in all areas of clinical human intervention. Perhaps there will be an increased development of majors or even master's/doctoral degrees in MindBody medicine.
5. States will consider the development of legal regulation or creation of credentials for the practice of MindBody medicine, for example, development of state licensing laws or regulations spelling out the type of training needed and area of practice authorized for someone putting themselves out to the public as a "MindBody medicine practitioner."
6. Governments and institutions will offer an increase of grant monies to investigate and apply MindBody medicine, for example, money allocated to improve and expand research into the understanding, effectiveness, and appropriate application of MindBody interventions.

7. Insurers will appreciate the cost-effectiveness of MindBody medicine and begin covering these interventions under their insurance plans. As we learn more about the effectiveness of MindBody interventions, it will be more evident that paying for a MindBody intervention is good economics. For example, since we know that some people can use visual imagery to enhance their immune system, then why not pay for that training as part of a treatment requiring enhanced immunity?
8. There will be increased application of all MindBody interventions, especially hypnosis and neurofeedback. These are two powerful tools that have been neglected in general medical practice and offer promise for a variety of problems. For example, hypnosis can be more widely applied in pediatrics, anesthesia, and wound healing. In fact, its many known applications (mentioned in Chapter 1) have yet to be utilized as fully as needed. Neurofeedback (a type of biofeedback) will bring more and more results with behavioral problems and will improve the volitional control of thoughts toward a body system or disease to enhancing healing.
9. We will continue to learn more about enhancing wellness using MindBody interventions. This will result in an emphasis on the development of wellness in people rather than the treatment of illness. This is following a current trend in psychology to focus on developing wellness (Bosnak, 2002; Seligman, Steen, et al., 2005); the application of MindBody interventions to help people have richer, more fulfilled existences. For example, the focus will shift from curing a disease to helping someone be more well integrated as a person with a healthful sense of security, sense of self-esteem, and sense of fulfillment and be better able to relate positively to others.

SUGGESTED READING

Bosnak, K. (May 2–4 2002). *Use of dreams for physical health.* Report presented at Harvard's program in science and MindBody medicine, Cambridge, MA.

Kenney, J. W. (2000). Women's "inner-balance": A comparison of stressors, personality traits and health problems by age groups. *Journal of Advanced Nursing, 31*, 639–650.

Seligman, M.E., Steen, T., et al. (2005). Positive psychology progress: Empirical validation of interventions. *American Psychologist, 60*, 410–421. [Dr. Seligman and his colleagues are bringing this concept into the research arena.]

Appendix A

Definitions of the Mind

WHAT IS THE MIND?

When it comes to defining *mind*, we discover a variety of thinking that results in many definitions and ideas regarding its definition and description. These definitions and ideas range from mind as spirit (Aristotle) to mind as matter (Locke). They also go from mind as individual (Rene Descartes) to mind as universal (Larry Dossy). If we are going to study this phenomenon of MindBody medicine, then it will be helpful to consider some definitions of and ideas about mind from a variety of thinkers. Before continuing, we suggest you review your thoughts on the subject of mind. As you review the following definitions and ideas, critically compare them to your thoughts on this subject.

We arranged this appendix to provide you a quick visual reference. Each number is followed by the definition or idea and then a list of the thinkers who have put forth that definition or idea. For further investigation, we include in parentheses the titles of the original work in which the ideas are found.

DEFINITIONS/IDEAS ON THE TOPIC OF "THE MIND"

1. The mind is the human consciousness that originates in the brain and is manifested especially in thought, perception, feeling, will, memory or imagination (*American Heritage Dictionary*).
2. The mind is the faculty of the soul for thinking and judging.*
   Aristotle (*Physics, On the Soul, Ethics, Politics*)
   Plato (*Republic, Timaeus, Theaetetus*)
   Plotinus (*First* and *Third Ennead*)
   Augustine (*Confessions, City of God*)
   Aquinas (*Summa Theologica*)
   Epictetus (*The Discourses*)
   Dante (*The Divine Comedy*)
3. The mind is the directing principle of the soul.*
   Lucretius (*The Nature of Things*)

4. The mind is equal to the soul and is identical with thinking.*
   Descartes (*Discourses, Meditations*)
5. The mind is presented as a particular mode of that attribute of God which is thought.*
   Spinoza (*Ethics*)
6. The mind is intelligence or self-consciousness, knowing itself as universal: the unity of intellect and will.*
   Hagel (*Philosophy of Right, Philosophy of History*)
7. The mind is the functioning of the intellect: the acts of understanding, judgment, and reason.*
   Francis Bacon (*Advancement of Learning, Novum Organum*)
8. The mind equals the unity of mental function (i.e., sensing, understanding, reasoning).*
   Immanuel Kant (*Discourse on Pure Reason*)
9. The mind is the totality of mental processes.*
   William James (*Psychology*)
   Freud (Interpretation of Dreams, Unconscious, General Introduction to Psychoanalysis)
10. The mind is a self-reflective information processor.
    Ernest Rossi and David Cheek (*Mind-Body Therapy: Methods of Ideodynamic Healing in Hypnosis*)
11. The mind is what the brain does.
    Carl Sagan (*Cosmos*)
12. The mind is the flow of information as it moves about the cells, organs, and systems of the body.
    Candice Pert (*Molecules of Emotions*)
13. The mind is fundamental to the world but not the exclusive property of the physical body (i.e., mind is universal).
    Larry Dossey (*Reinventing Medicine*)
14. Our definition is that the mind is the capability to perform cognitive functions. In humans, the mind is the energy within every living cell of our body. We use the brain (an anatomical tool) to govern this energy.

SUGGESTED READING

Carpenter, A. (1998). *Kant's earliest solution to the mind/body problem.* Unpublished doctoral dissertation, University of California at Berkley. Retrieved from: http://www.andrewcarpenter.net/diss/diss_pdf_.html.

Dossey, L. (1999). *Reinventing Medicine*. San Francisco: Harper.

Harth, E. *The Creative Loop: How the Brain Makes a Mind*. Reading, MA: Addison-Wesley.

Hinrichs, B. (1998). Computing the mind: A scientific approach to the philosophy of mind and brain. *The Humanist, 58,* 28–30.

Lloyd, A.J. (2004). A Toolbox for humanity: More than 9000 years of thought. *The Great Books of the Western World*. Encyclopedia Britannica.

Kant, I. (1998). Critique of Pure Reason (P. Guyer, Trans.). In P. Guyer and A. W. Wood (Eds.), *The Cambridge Edition of the Works of Immanuel Kant*. Cambridge, UK: Cambridge University Press.

Pert, C. (1997). *Molecules of Emotion*. New York: Scribner.

Rossi, E., & Cheek, D. (1998). *Mind-Body Therapy: Methods of Ideodynamic Healing in Hypnosis*. New York: Norton.

Sagan, C. (1985) *Cosmos*. New York: Ballantine Books

*__Note:__ The works cited by numbers 2 through 9 are considered classics in Western literature. They may be found as a number of editions by many publishers. The best quick reference is *The Great Ideas of the Western World*, published by Encyclopedia Britannica. (Lloyd, A.J. (2004). A Toolbox for humanity: More than 9000 years of thought. *The Great Books of the Western World*. Encyclopedia Britannica.)

Appendix B

Effectiveness of MindBody Medicine

AIDS

	Intervention	Results	References
1	Forty patients prayed for 1 hour/day, 6 days a week for 10 weeks (experimental group)	Experimental group had fewer AIDS-related illnesses; illnesses they had were less severe, required fewer hospitalizations and fewer days in the hospital	Sicher et al. (1998)
2	Stress management	Slowed rate of decline in immunological cells	Autonie (1995)
3	CBT	Slow progression of infection by improving immune system's ability to control herpes type 2 virus	Lutgendorf (1997)

Anxiety: Obsessive-Compulsive Disorder

	Intervention	Results	References
1	10 weeks of CBT	Decrease in symptoms, with 70% improvement; results similar to medication	Schwarts (1996)
2	Meditation	Significant lowering	Speca & Carlson (2000)

Anxiety: General Anxiety Disorder

	Intervention	Results	References
1	Meditation	Reduced anxiety Decrease in muscle tension	Schneider et al. (1995); Kabat-Zinn et al. (1992); Brown (2003); NCCAM (1999); Speca & Carlson (2000) Mayo Clinic
2	Psychotherapy	Reduced anxiety	Barlow (1996)
3	Hypnosis	Reduced feelings of anxiety	Barlow (1996)
4	Energy focus	Elimination of some phobias	Gallo (1998)

Arthritis

	Intervention	Outcome	References
1	Support group (12 sessions over a 6-week period)	Decrease in pain by 10%; saved $75 per patient per year	Lorig, Mazonso, Holman, & Mazonson (1993)
2	Expressive writing (i.e., freely associating in a narrative form, expressing both affect and cognition on topics relating to stressful experiences)	Improved range of motion and reduced symptoms	Smyth et al. (1999)
3	Prayer	Prayed-for group had less pain and better mobility	Mathews et al. (2002)

Asthma

	Intervention	Outcome	References
1	Group education and support	49% decrease in acute visits for treatment	Wilson et al. (1993)
2	Relaxation training	Relaxation of airways	Lehrer (1998)
3	Yoga	Minimized symptoms	Vedanthan et al. (1998)
4	Expressive writing	Symptom reduction	LaPuma (1999)

Bleeding

	Intervention	Outcome	References
1	Hypnosis	Stopped blood flow	Bennet & Benan (1985)
2	Energy focus	Decrease in healing time	Wirth (1990); L. Dossey (1999)

Cancer

	Intervention	Outcome	References
1	Meditation	Lower distress and anxiety in cancer patients	Speca & Carlson (2000)
2	Imagery	Shrinking of tumors	Dossey (1999); Siegal (2003)
3	Group therapy	Improvement in mood and extended life spread	Classen & Spregal (1989); Fawzy & Fawzy (1993); Dittmann (2003); Classen et al. (2001); Cunningham & Tocco (1989); Cain et al. (1986); Richardson et al. (1990)

Cardiovascular: Heart

	Intervention	Outcome	References
1	Stress management	Reduced risk of recurrence	Blumental et al. (1997)
2	Prayer daily for 4 weeks for speedy recovery by five Christian volunteers	Better outcome than control (i.e., decreased need for medicine and additional procedures and less time in hospital)	Harris (1999)
3	Prayer (daily)	Five times less need for antibiotics; three times less likely to develop pulmonary edema than control group	Byrd (1988)
4	Meditation	Prevention of heart attack and stroke	Castillo-Richmond & Schneider (2002)

Cardiovascular: Hypertension

	Intervention	Outcome	References
1	Meditation	Lowered BP in hypertensive individuals	NCCAM (1999); Barnes (1999, 2003), text page 16; Psychosomatic Research
2	Psychotherapy	Reduction of both systolic and diastolic BP; decrease in diastolic BP and mean arterial pressure	Linden (1994); Schneider (1995); Lawler (2003)
3	Yoga: hatha yoga practice for 1 hour per day	Normalized high BP	Sung Dell et al. (2000)
4	Biofeedback	Lowered BP in hypertensive individuals controlled evaluation of thermal biofeedback in treatment of elevated blood pressure in unmedicated mild hypertension	Canino, Cordona, et al. (1994); Nako, Nomaron, et al. (1997); Blanchard, Eisele, Vollmer, Payne, Gordon, Cornish, Gilmore (1996)
5	Music therapy	Lowered BP in hypertensive individuals	Gaynos (2000)

Carpal Tunnel Syndrome

Intervention	Outcome	References
Yoga	Reduction in pain	Garfinkel et al. (1999)

Childbirth

	Intervention	Outcome	References
1	Emotional support during labor and reassurance	Labor length decreased 25%; odds of cesarean section decreased 34%; odds of needing analgesia decreased 23%	Klaus (1992)
2	Prepartum training in relaxation	Women who receive prepartum training in relaxation, need fewer visits to their health care providers	Kennel (1991); Klaus (1992)
3	Hypnosis	Conversion of breech presentation	Mehl (1994)

Depression

	Intervention	Outcome	References
1	Support groups	Decrease in loneliness that related to depression	*National Psychologist (2003)*
2	Writing of poetry in therapy	Reduced depression.	Lapore (1997)
3	Meditation	Reduced depression.	Segal (2000)Brown (2003)
4	Psychotherapy	Reduced symptoms and depression; reductions lasted longer than with medications alone as effective as medicine	Keller (2000)Antonuccio (1994)Depression Panel of NIH (1993)
5	Psychotherapy	Improvement is comparable to pharmacotherapy	Robinson et al. (1990)
6	Psychotherapy CBT	As effective as medication	Ruske, Blecke, & Reinfraw (2006)
7	Psychotherapy CBT	As effective as light therapy for seasonal affective disorder	Rohan (2004)
8	CBT interpersonal therapy with medications	Response was faster than with medicine alone	Thase & Howland (1994)Fava, Grandi. Zielezny, et al. (1994)Thase, Greenhouse, Franke, et al. (1997)

Diabetes

	Intervention	Outcome	References
1	Progressive muscle relaxation	Lower blood sugar	Swartz (2004)
2	Support groups	Saved hospital $2,319 per patient treated; decreased hospital visits by 73%; decreased hospital stay by 78%	Report from Harvard and University of Southern California Medical Center

Gastrointestinal System

	Intervention	Outcome	References
	Hypnosis	Improvement in functional dyspepsia	Calvert (2002)

Immune System

	Intervention	Outcome	References
1	Imagery	Increase in lymphocyte count and enhancement of natural killer cells; change in individual lymphocyte count; shrinking of cancer tumors	Kiecolt-Glasser et al. (1985); Achterberg (1993); L. Dossey (1999); Siegal (2003)
2	Humor/laughter	Increased natural killer cells and decreased stress hormones	Beck & Tan (1996)

Insomnia

	Intervention	Outcome	References
1	Meditation	Improvement in sleep patterns	NIH Fields of Practice (1999)
2	Psychotherapy	Reduction of insomnia	Morin et al. (1999); Jacob (2004); Palson (2006)
3	Cognitive-behavioral psychotherapy	Effective in improving sleep time and sleep quality	Smith & Rerbeck (2006)
4	Humor/laughter	Increased length of pain-free sleep	Hutchinson (2003)

Irritable Bowel Syndrome

	Intervention	Outcome	References
1	Hypnosis	Reduction in distress and number of visits to physician	Peter Whorell, M.D., gastroenterologist William Whitehead, Ph.D., professor, Johns Hopkins
2	Psychotherapy—superior or equal to medicine (i.e., brief psychodynamic hypnosis)	Control the condition better than antispasmodics and bulk agents for up to 2 years of therapy	Blanchard (1996); Malamood, Howard, M.D. Professional Psychology: Research and Practice; June
3	Cognitive-behavioral psychotherapy	Improvement of symptoms	Palson (2006)
4	CBT and medication	Stabilized condition with significant reduction in symptoms and superior to medicines alone	Hymann (2000); Read (1999)
5	Biofeedback	Stabilized or eliminated condition	Schwartz & Andrasick (2006)

Menopause

	Intervention	Outcome	References
1	Four 1-hour sessions over 6 to 8 weeks learning muscular relaxation and deep-breathing techniques	Reduced frequency of hot flashes by 50%; 91% rated themselves improved after 3 minutes; 25% had no hot flashes; all compared to control	Hunter & Liao (1995)
2	Positive self-talk	Reduced frequency of hot flashes	Hunter & Liao (1995)

Pain

	Intervention	Outcome	References
1	Imagery	Reduction/elimination of pain	Melzak (1990), see page 11; Keuckenboom (1988); Rossman (1993); Meyer (1995)
2	Meditation	Reduction of chronic pain	Kabat-Zinn et al. (1998); Caudill et al. (1991); NIH Fields of Practice (1999)
3	Psychotherapy	Helped in pain management; effective in modifying lower back pain	Winterowed, Beck, et al. (2003); Van Talden et al. (2000)
4	No intervention breathing techniques	Airway clearance in bronchiectasis	Patterson (2004)
5	Music therapy	Reduction of pain	Gaynos (2000)
6	Energy focus	Decreased or eliminated perception of pain	Keller (1993)
7	Biofeedback	Elimination of headache pain and frequency	Sarafine (2000)

Panic Disorder

	Intervention	Outcome	References
1	Hypnosis	Worked better than medication in the long term	Barlow (2000); Coallow (1999)
2	CBT	Better than medication in the long term	Barlow (1996)
3	Yoga (Iyenger)	Reduced stress and physical pain	Garfinkel et al. (1999); Rush (1996)
4	Positive self-talk	Eliminated and decreased pain sensation	Chen (2000); Barlow (1996)

Psoriasis

	Intervention	Outcome	References
1	Biofeedback	Reduction in severity and recurrence	Goodman (1994); Polenghi (1994)
2	Mindfulness meditation	Enhance improvement	Kabat-Zinn (2000); Polenhi (1994)
3	Psychotherapy	Reduction of symptoms	Crossbart (1993)

REFERENCES

Stress

	Intervention	Outcome	References
1	Meditation	Significant lowering of stress and anxiety	Speca & (2000); Miller, Fletcher, et al. (1995); Ospina-Kummerer & Dixon (2001)
2	Expressive writing psychotherapy	Relieved stress	Eng, Fitzmaurice, et al. (2003)
3	Humor/Laughter	Reduction in stress levels	Bennett et al. (2003); Martin (2003)
4	Hypnosis	Reduced/eliminated stress	Bryant (2005); Butler (2005)

Temperomandibular Disorder

Intervention	Outcome	References
Hypnosis	Eliminated disorder or minimized discomfort	NIM-OAM Panel (May 1998)

Urinary Disorders

Intervention	Outcome	References
Biofeedback	Controls or illuminates urinary incontinence	Schwartz & Andrasick (2006)

Decrease in Use of Medical Services

	Intervention	Outcome	References
1	Psychotherapy	Decrease in use of medical procedures	Hiratsuka (1990)
2	Marital therapy	Decrease in use of medical system, resulting in financial savings	Crane (1997)

Achterberg, J., & Rider, M.S. (1993). The effects of music mediated imagery on neutrophils and lymphocytes. *Biofeedback and Self Regulation, 14*, 247–257.

Antonuccio, D.O., Danton, W.G., DeNelsky, G.Y., Greenberg, R.P., & Gordon, J.S. (1994). Raising questions about antidepressants. *Psychotherapy and psychosomatics, 68* (1), 3–14.

Autonie, M. (1995). Cited in *Monitor of the American Psychological Association.*

Barlow, D., Gorman, J.M., Shear, M.K., & Woods, S.W. (2000). Cognitive-behavioral therapy, imipramine, or their combination for panic disorder: A randomized controlled trial. *Journal of the American Medical Association, 283*, 2529–2536

Barlow, D.H. (1996). Advances in psychosocial treatment of anxiety disorders. *Archives of General Psychiatry, 53*, 727–735.

Beck, A.T., & Tan, S. (1996). Report on psychoneuroimmunology. *Research Society Meeting.*

Bennet, H., & Benan, D.R.. (1985). *Journal of Anesthesiology.*

Bennett, M.P., Zeller, J.M., Rosenberg, L., & McCann, J. (2003). The effect of mirthful laughter on stress and natural killer cell activity. Alternative *Therapies in Health and Medicine, 9*, 38–45.

Blanchard, E.B., Eisele, G., Vollmer, A., Payne, A., Gordon, M., Cornish, P., & Gilmore, L. (1996). Controlled evaluation of thermal biofeedback in treatment of elevated blood pressure in unmedicated mild hypertension. *Biofeedback Self Regulation Psychological Treatment of Irritable Syndrome, 21*(2), 167–190.

Blanchard, E., & Malamood, H.S. (1996). Psychological treatment, irritable bowel syndrome. *Professional Psychology; Research and Practice.*

Blanchard, E.B. & Malamood, H.S. (1996). Psychological treatment of irritable bowel syndrome. *American Psychological Association, 27*(3), 241–244.

Blumenthal, J.A., Jiang, W., Babyak, M.A., Krantz, D.S., Frid, D.J., Coleman, R.E., Waugh, R., Hanson, M., Appelbaum, M., O'Connor, C., & Morris, J.J. (1997). Stress management and exercise training cardiac patients with myocardial ischemia. *Archives of Internal Medicine, 157*, 2213–2223.

Brown, K.W., Moskowitz, D.S., (1997). Does unhappiness make you sick? The role of affect and neuroticism in the experience of common physical symptoms. *Journal of Personality, 72* (4), 907–917.

Butler, I.D. (2005). Hypnosis reduces distress and duration of an invasive medical procedure for children. *Pediatrics, 115* (1), 77–85.

Bryant, R.A., Moulds, M.I., Guthrie, R.M., & Nixon, R.D. (2005). The additive benefit of hypnosis and cognitive behavioral therapy in treating acute stress disorder. *Journal Consult Clinical Psychology, 73* (2), 334–340.

Byrd, R. (1988). Positive therapeutic effects of intercessory prayer in a coronary care population. *Southern Medicine Journal, 18.*

Cain, E. N., et al. (1986). Psychosocial benefits of a cancer support group. *Cancer, 57*, 183–189.

Calvert, E.L., Houghton, L.A., Cooper, P., Morris, J., Whorwell, P.J. (2002). Long-term improvement in functional dyspepsia using hypnotherapy. Gastroenterology, 123 (6), 1778–1785.

Canino, E., Cardona, R., Monsalve, P., Perez Acuna, F., Lopez, B., & Fragachan, F. (1994). A behavioral treatment program as a therapy in the control of primary hypertension. *Acta Cient Venen, 45*, 23–30.

Castillo-Richmond, & Schneider, R.H. (2002). Effects of stress reduction on carotid aterioscierosis in hypertensive African Americans. *Stroke, 31*, 568.

Caudill, M., et al. (1991). Decreased clinical use by chronic pain patients responding to behavioral medicine interventions. *The Journal of Chronic Pain, 7,* 305.

Chen, E.J.M. (2000). Behavioral and cognitive interventions in the treatment of pain in children. *Pediatric Clinics of North America, 47,* 513-25..

Classen, C., et al. (2001). Supportive-expressive group therapy and distress in patients with metastatic breast cancer. A randomized clinical intervention trial. *Archives of General Psychiatry,* 58, 494–501.

Crane, D.R. (1997). Why marital therapy matters: The economic and social consequences of divorce. In *Fundamentals of Marital Therapy.* New York: Brunner/Mazel.

Grossbart, T. (1993). The skin matters of the flesh. In D. Goleman (Ed.). *Mind Body Medicine.* Yonkers, NY: Consumer Reports Books.

Cunningham, A.J., & Tocco, E.K. (1989). A randomized trial of group psychoeducational therapy for cancer patients. *Patient Education and Counseling, 14,* 101–114.

Dittmann, M. (2003). Coping with cancer through social connection. *Monitor on Psychology, 34* (3)24–26.

Dossey, B. M., Keegan, L., & Guzzetta, C.E. (2000). *Holistic Nursing.* Gaithersburg, MD: Aspen Publishers.

Dossey, L. (1999). *Reinventing Medicine: Beyond Mind Body to a New Area of Healing.* San Francisco: Harper.

Eng, P.M., Fitzmaurice, G., Kubzansky, L.D., Rimm, E.B., & Kawachi. (2003). Anger expression and risk of coronary artery disease among male health professionals. *Psychosomatic Medicine, 65,* 100–110.

Fava, G., Grandi, S., Zielezny, M., et al. (1994). Cognitive behavioral treatment of residual symptoms in primary major depressive disorder. *American Journal of Psychiatry, 151,* 1295–1299

Fawzy, F.I. (1995). Critical review of psychosocial intervention and cancer care. *Archives of General Psychiatry, 52,* 100–1300.

Fawzy & Fawzy. (1993). Malignant melanoma. *Archives of General Psychiatry, 50,* 681–689.

Gallo, F. (1998). *Energy Psychology.* Boca Raton, FL: CRC Press.

Garfinkel, M.S., Singhal, A., Katz, W.A., et al. (1998). Yoga-based intervention for carpal tunnel syndrome: A randomized controlled trial. *Journal of the American Medical Association, 280*(18), 1601–1603.

Gaynor, L.M. (2000). Sounds of healing: A physician reveals the therapeutic power of sound, voice, and music. Broadway Books.

Goodman, M. (1994). An hypothesis explaining the successful treatment of psoriasis with thermal biofeedback. *Biofeedback Self Regulation, 19,* 347–352.

Grossbart, T. (1993). The skin matters of the flesh. In D. Goleman (Ed.), *Mind Body-Medicine,* pp. 145-175, Yonkers, NY: Consumer Reports Books.

Harris, W.S., Gowda, M., Kolb, J.W., Strychacz, C.P., Vacek, J.L., Jones, P.G., Forker, A., O'Keefe, J.H., & McCalliste. (1999). A randomized, controlled trial of the effects of remote, intercessory prayer on outcomes in patients admitted to the coronary care unit. *Archives of Internal Medicine, 159,* 2273–2278.

Hiratsuka, J. (1990). Brief mental health care can reduce medical bill, four-year study confirms. *NASW News, 35.*

Hunter, M.S., & Liao, K.L.M. (March 1995). *Evaluation of a four session cognitive behavioral intervention for menopausal hot flashes.* Paper presented at British Psychological Society annual conference.

Hutchinson, L. (2003). Taking humor seriously–Ha. *Paradigm, 19.*

Hymann, M., Heymann-Monnikes, I., Arnold, R., Florin, I., Herda, C., Melfsen, S., & Monnikes, H. (2000). The combination of medical treatment plus multi-component behavioral therapy is superior to medical treatment alone in the treatment of irritable bowel syndrome. *American Journal of Gastroenterology,* 95 (4), 981–999.

Jacob, G.D. (2004). Cognitive behavior therapy and pharmacotherapy for insomnia: a randomized control trial and direct comparison. *Archives of Internal Medicine, 164,* 1888–1896.

Kwekkenboom, K., et al. (1998). Imaging ability and effective use of guided imagery. *Research in Nurse Health, 21,* 189–198.

Kabat-Zinn, J. (1986). Four-year follow up of a meditation based program for the self-regulation of chronic pain. *Clinical Journal of Pain 2,* 150–173.

Kabat-Zinn, J. (2000). Report of annual Harvard Scientific Conference on Alternative Medicine. *Psychosomatic Medicine, 60,* 625–632.

Kabat-Zinn, J., et al. (1992). Effectiveness of a meditation based stress reduction program in the treatment of anxiety disorders. *American Journal of Psychology, 149,* 936–994.

Kabat-Zinn, J., et al. (1998). Influence of a mindfulness meditation-based stress reduction intervention on rates of skin clearing in patients with moderate to severe psoriasis undergoing phototherapy and photochemotherapy. *Psychosomatic Medicine, 60,* 625–632.

Keller, E. (1993). *The effects of therapeutic touch on tension headache pain.* Master's thesis, University of Missouri, Columbia.

Kiecolt-Glaser, J.K. Glaser, R., Williger, D., Stout, J., Messick, (1985). Psycho-social enhancement of immunocompetence in a geriatric population. *Health Psychology, 4,* 25–29.

Kennell, J., Klaus, M., McGrath, S., Robertson, S., & Hinkley, C. (1992). Psychological support during childbirth. *Jordemodern, 105*(9), 308–310.

Lapore, S.J. (1997). Expressive writing moderates the relation between intrusive thoughts and depressive symptoms. *Journal of Personality and Social Psychology, 73,* 1030–1039.

Lawler, K.A., Younger, J.W., Piferi, R.L., Billington, E., Jobe, R., Edmondson, K., & Jones, W.H. (2003). A change of heart: Cardiovascular correlates of forgiveness in response to interpersonal conflict. *Journal of Behavioral Medicine, 26* (5), 373–393.

Lehrer, P.M, (1998). Emotionally triggered asthma: a review of research literature and some hypotheses for self regulation therapies. *Application Psychophysical Biofeedback,* March 23, 13–41.

LaPuma. (June 1999). Writing therapy to reduce asthma and RA symptoms. *Alternative Medicine Alert,* 2, 82–83.

Linden, W.C. (1994). Clinical effectiveness of non-drug treatment for hypertension, a meta-analysis. *Annals of Behavioral Medicine, 16,* 35–45.

Lorig, K.R., Mazonso, P.D., Holman, H.R., & Mazonson. (1993). Evidence suggesting that health education for self management in patients with chronic arthritis has sustained health benefits while reducing health care costs. *Arthritis and Rheumatoid Arthritis, 36,* 439–446.

Lutgendorf, S.K., Michael, H.A., Gail, I., Klimas, N., Fletcher, M.N. & Schneiderman, N. (1997). Cognitive processing style, mood, and immune function following HIV seropositivity notification. *Cognitive Therapy and Research, 21* (2), 157–184.

Martin, R.A. (2003). Humor and their relation to psychological well-being: Development of the humor styles. *Journal of Research in Personality, 37* (1).

Matthews, D.A., Marlowe, S.M., & MacNutt, F.S. (2000). Effects of intercessory prayer on patients with rheumatoid arthritis. *Southern Medical Journal, 93* (12), 1177–1186.

Mehl, L. (1994). Hypnosis and conversion of the breech to the vertex presentation. *Archives of Family Medicine, 3*, 881–887.

Melzak, R. (1990). The tragedy of needless pain. *Scientific American, 262*, 27–33.

Meyers, T.J., & Mark, M.M. (1995). Effects of psychosocial interventions on adult cancer patients. A meta-analysis of randomized experiments. *Health Psychology*, 14, 101–108.

Miller, J., Fletcher, K., & Kabat-Zinn, J. (1995). Three-year follow-up and clinical implications of a mindfulness meditation-based stress reduction intervention in the treatment of anxiety disorders. *General Hospital Psychiatry, 17*, 192–200.

Morin, C.M., et al. (1999). A randomized controlled trial of stress reduction for hypertension in older African Americans. *Hypertension, 6*, 820–827.

Nako, M., Nomaron, S., et al. (1997). Clinical effects of blood pressure biofeedback treatment on hypertension by auto shaping. *Psychosomatic Medicine, 59*, 331–338.

NIH Fields of Practice. (November 1999). National Institutes of Health Web site. Retrieved from: http://nccam.nib.gov/ncccom/what-is-cam/fields/mind.htm#meditation.

Ospina-Kammerer, V., & Dixon, D.R. (2001). Coping with burnout: Family physicians and family social workers—what do they have in common? *Journal of Family Social Work, 5*(4), 85–93.

Palson, O. (2006). The nature of IBS and the need for a psychological approach. *International Journal of Clinical and Experimental Hypnosis; 54*, 1–5.

Patterson, J.E., Bradley, J.M., Elborn, J.S. (2004). Airway clearance in bronchiectasis: A randomized crossover trial of active cycle of breathing techniques (incorporating postural drainage and vibration) versus test of incremental respiratory endurance. *Chronic Respiratory Disorders 2004, 1*(3), 127–130.

Polenghi, M.M. (1994). Experience with psoriasis in psychosomatic dermatology clinic. *Acta Derm Venarol Supplement (Stockholm), 86*, 65–66.

Richardson, J.L., et al. (1990). Support group. *Journal of Clinical Oncology, 8*, 356–364.

Robinson, L.A., et al. (1990). Psychotherapy for the treatment of depression: Comparison review of outcome research. *Psychological Bulletin*.

Rohan, K.J., Lindsey, K.T., Roecklein, K.A., Lacy, T.J. (2004). Cognitive-behavioral therapy, light therapy, and their combination in treating seasonal affective disorder. *Journal of Affective Disorder, 80* (2-3), 273–283.

Rossman, M. (1993). Imagery: Learning to use the mind's eye. In D. Goleman (Ed.), *Mind Body Medicine*. Yonkers, New York: Consumer Reports Books.

Rush, A.J. (1996). The role of psychotherapy in the treatment of depression: review of two practice guidelines. *Arch Gen Psychiatry, 53* (4), 298-300.

Ruske, S., Blecke, D., & Reinfraw, M. (2006). Cognitive therapy for depression. *American Family Physician, 73.*

Rush, A. (1996). *The Modern Book of Yoga: Exercising Mind, Body, and Spirit.* New York: Bantam Dell.

Sarafine, E. (2000). Age comparison in acquiring biofeedback control and success in reducing headache pain. *Annals of Behavior Medicine, 2,* 10.

Schwarts, J. (1996). Psychotherapy as strong as drug treatment for obsessive compulsive disorder. *Archives of General Psychiatry.*

Schwartz, M., & Andrasick, F. (2006). *Biofeedback: A Practitioner's Guide.* New York: Guilford Press.

Segal. (2002). *Meaningfulness Based Cognitive Therapies for Depression.* New York: Guilford Press.

Sicher, F. Targ, E., Moore, D., & Smith, H.S. (1998). A randomized double blind study of two effects of distance healing in a population with advanced AIDS. *Western Journal of Medicine, 169,* 6.356–6.363.

Siegal, B. (2003). Healing our lives. *Advances, 19,* 13–14.

Smith, M., & Rerbeck. (2006). Who is a candidate for cognitive behavioral therapy for insomnia. *Health Psychology; 25,* 15–19.

Speca, M., & Carlson, L. (2000). How do you feel about cancer now? *Psychosomatic Medicine, 62.*

Spiegel, D. (1995). Support group. *Public Health Reports, 110,* 298.

Sung Dell, R.H., et al. (2000). *American Journal of Hypertension, 13,* 185A–186A.

Swartz, R. (2004). *The Mind-Body Diabetes Revelation.* New York: Free Press.

Symth, J.M., et al. (1999). *Effect of Writing About Stressful Experiences on Symptom Reduction in Patients with Asthma and Rheumatoid Arthritis.*

Thase, M.E., Greenhouse, J.B., Franke, E., et al. (1997). Treatment of major depression with psychotherapy, pharmacotherapy, psychotherapy combinations, or pharmacotions. *Archives of General Psychiatry, 54,* 1009–1015.

Thase, M.E., & Howland, R.H. (1994). Refractory depression: Relevance of psychosocial factors and therapies. *Psychiatry Annals, 24,* 232–240.

Van Talden, M.W., et al. (2000). Analysis of research. *Spine, 26,* 270–281.

Vedanthan, P.R., et al. (1998). Clinical study of yoga techniques in university students with asthma. A controlled study. *Allergy Asthma Procedure,* 19, 3–9.

Whitehead, W.E. (1992). Behavioral medicine approaches to gastrointestinal disorders, *Journal of Consulting and Clinical Psychology, 60,* 605–612.

Wilson et al. (1993). *American Journal of Medicine* from American Institute for Research at Kaiser.

Winterowed, C., Beck, A., et al. (2003). *Cognitive Therapy With Chronic Pain Patients.* New York: Springer.

Wirth, D. (1990). The effect of non-contact therapeutic touch on the healing rate of full-thickness surgical wounds. *Subtle Energies, 1,* 1–20.

Appendix C

Deeper Understanding of Stress

DEFINITIONS

The following terms are important in understanding stress:

Burnout: The syndrome of emotional exhaustion and cynicism that frequently occurs among people who do people work, that is, who spend considerable time in close encounters with other people (Maslach, 1976).

Stress: Stress is an adaptive response mediated by individual characteristics or psychological processes; that is, it is a consequence of any external action, situation, or event that places special physical or psychological demands on a person (Ivancevich & Matteson, 1981). From the individual's point of view, stress lies between the stressor (event) and the subjective experience or reactions to the event (Breznitz & Goldberger, 1993).

Stressors (event): We use *stressors* interchangeably with *event*.

Stress reactions (stress): We use *stress reactions* interchangeably with *stress*.

Coping: Cognitive and behavioral efforts to manage stressful encounters that individuals appraise as taxing personal resources. Lazarus and Folkman (in Schafer, 1996, p. 324) define coping as constantly changing cognitive and behavioral efforts to manage specific external or internal demands that are appraised as taxing or exceeding the resources of the person (in Schafer, 1996, p. 324).

Positive coping or **adaptive coping:** Dealing effectively with stressors in life; having a range of options available to deal with stressful events.

Negative coping or **maladaptive coping:** This form of coping results in unnecessary distress for the person dealing ineffectively with stressors in life (Schafer, 1996, p. 327).

A theoretical framework is the basis for a research study. There is no one theory at the present time that includes all approaches to stress and burnout. The current literature mentions three conceptual models: (1)

stress theory, (2) biospychosocial models, and (3) models of family stress and coping.

Stress theory: Previous work was stimulated to a great extent by classic animal studies of Selye (1936a, 1936b, 1937, 1946; Collip, 1936). In 1936, Seyle formulated a definition of stress as "the nonspecific (that is, common) result of any demand upon the body" (p. vii), be it a mental or a somatic demand for survival and the accomplishment of our aims. At that time, only three objective indicators were recognized no matter how stress was produced. These indicators were "the mobilization of the anterior pituitary-adrenal axis, the readily observable involution of the thymico-lymphatic system and the appearance of peptic ulcers" (p. viii). To understand a scientist's point of view and to make use of stress theory, Selye's philosophical paradigm needs to be highlighted:

1. Stress is nonspecific. This does not mean that all stress situations are identical because stress is never seen in isolation.
2. A stressor is whatever produces stress, with or without functioning hormonal or nervous systems. This could be a somatic demand such as the healing of a wound or resistance to infection. It could also be putting up with an intolerable partner at work. Selye in 1937 constructed experiments on stress reaction and the entire general adaptation syndrome (GAS) mainly from the viewpoint of the hormonal system. His research results showed that, even in totally hypophysectomized or adrenalectomized rats, exposure to stress produces all the stereotyped nonspecific responses characteristic of demands as such, except those made by stimuli that are relayed through the pituitary-adrenocortical axis. The importance of corticotropin-releasing factor or even adrenocorticotropic hormone (ACTH) is still debated, yet it is universally accepted that variations in corticotropin-releasing factor or ACTH production are the most reliable of the existence of a state of stress (p. ix).
3. Much confusion exists concerning various views on corticoid and ACTH feedback and corticoid utilization. There is no doubt that, under normal conditions, excess corticoid administration can diminish corticoid production through the inhibition of ACTH secretion. In addition, excessive amounts of ACTH will act on the pituitary and decrease ACTH production itself and thus, secondarily, decrease corticoid secretion.
4. The shift in pituitary activity during stress may be due to lowered receptivity of peripheral organs and a variety of other conditioning factors, such as species differences or significant variations, depending on the intensity and the duration of exposure.
5. A psychological stressor can act only if it is appreciated as such. Otherwise, there is no stress, no demand. For example, a person

under anesthesia cannot be placed under stress by even the most aggravating coworker.

6. A stressor is always accompanied by specific side effects; both internal and external predisposing or immunizing factors modify the response. These factors, such as previous exposure to stress, heredity, air pollution, tradition, education, and seasonal variations, are called *conditioning factors*.
7. There is a distinction between good stress and bad stress. Good stress is called *eustress* (*eu* = good), and bad stress is called *distress*; which is the detrimental variety.
8. Selye emphasized that stress is not a yes-or-no phenomenon. He indicated that stress can exist in various degrees and intensities and make different demands, which do not always equal stress reactions.
9. The stress diseases are also a matter of degree. For example, high blood pressure, heart attacks, mental breakdown, migraines, and insomnia are listed in this category, although additional factors likewise play a role. On the other hand, lethal bullet wounds and paralysis after complete transection of the spinal cord are consequences that may cause stress. The majority of all maladies for which the patient seeks medical attention are predominantly due to stress, especially psychogenic stress, which is the basis of psychosomatic medicine. In Selye's viewpoint, stress tests are useful only to the degree that they can be individualized. They are like computerized diagnoses or recommendations for therapy. Statistical methods and procedures are quite valid in that they show how most persons would behave under certain circumstances, but they say nothing about the individual patient because no individual is average. The closer a researcher can consider the whole patient, including the person's environment, the more precisely a diagnosis can be made. This is the basis of holistic medicine.
10. Selye makes a clear distinction between treatment techniques (e.g., biofeedback, relaxation, physical exercise) and a philosophy of life. He states that both are important, but that the greatest challenge to humanity at the present time is to find a philosophy of life, a code of behavior, that gives good guidance, not to avoid stress (for that is impossible), but to cope with it to achieve health, long life, and happiness (Selye, 1980, pp. v–xiii).

Building on Selye's theoretical model of stress, writers of the history of stress cite several early laboratory and clinical sources. The 19th century French physiologist Bernard (1879) enormously advanced the subject by pointing out that the internal environment of a living organism must remain fairly constant despite changes in the external environment. Bernard (1865) extended the Cartesian epistemology to legitimize the study of living things as physical entities. The German physiologist Pfluger (1877) indicated that there is a relationship between active adaptation and the steady state. The Belgian physiologist Fredericq (1885) expressed a similar view that the living organism compensates and neutralizes to repair any disturbance in the system.

In this century, the American physiologist Cannon (1939) introduced the term *homeostasis,* from the Greek *homoios,* meaning similar, and *stasis,* meaning position or staying power within the organism (Breznitz & Goldberger, 1993, pp. 3–17). Cannon's research was concerned with the specific mechanisms of change in the external environment while allowing for optimum bodily function. He described clearly that human beings can invoke behavioral changes to alter the environment or can use autonomic and endocrine mechanisms to alter metabolic and other bodily processes to regain optimal conditions (Lovallo, 1997).

To this list can be added Harold G. Wolff's experiments in psychosomatics and Dunbar's systematic organization of psychosomatics. Also add the epidemiological investigations of Holmes and Rahe and the development of the psychology of coping. In the early 1950s, stress research found a common ground in a systems approach to health and disease (Kugelman, 1992). Just as the theory about germs has served to inhibit relating psychosocial factors to infectious disease, the stress theory has to a great extent limited the entire field of psychosomatic research. As pointed out, each form of stimulation has both nonspecific and specific effects on the organism (Lazarus, 1974; Levi, 1974; Selye, 1973) demonstrated that certain levels of arousing stimuli are both necessary and beneficial to the organism. As Selye continued his experimentation in classical animal studies in 1946, he developed a theory of physiological adaptation. His theoretical framework, the GAS, linked environmental stress to a nonspecific adrenocortical response. The GAS has three stages: (1) alarm reaction, (2) resistance, and (3) exhaustion. Increased adrenocortical activity produces resistance. If severe and or prolonged stress exceeded the animal's ability to sustain sufficient adrenocortical secretion, adrenal cortex "exhaustion" occurred, which led to either disease or death (Plaut & Friedman, 1981).

Disease (dis-ease) can be viewed as any persistent, harmful disturbance of equilibrium within the body. Three subsystems in our body (nervous, endocrine, and immune) maintain this equilibrium. To illustrate the interface between psychology and the immune system, Borysenko (1991) defined stress as the perception of threat to the physical or psychological well-being and the perception that these individual responses are inadequate to cope with it. He presented an overview of the interface between psychology and the immune system.

The fight-or-flight response is elicited in acute stress, resulting in increased sympathetic nerve activity and release of epinephrine (adrenaline). These physiological changes are short. The GAS is elicited in chronic stress and involves pituitary-induced corticosteroid release. The sympathetic nervous system is always active. It plays an essential role in the body's adjustments to normal demands in concert with the parasympathetic nervous system, and it is essential for the integration and expression of the fight-flight response during times of stress. The parasympathetic nervous system sends fibers to its target organs by way of the cranial nerves arising from the brain stem and by way of the sacral segment of the spinal cord. The parasympathetic division generally supports feeding, energy storage, and reproduction.

The body secretes catecholamines, stress hormones. The primary stress hormones are epinephrine and cortisol. The medulla of the adrenal gland is activated by sympathetic preganglionic fibers; in response, it secretes the catecholamine epinephrine into the systemic circulation. During stressful periods, the epinephrine secretion increases. Cortisol, the second major stress hormone, is capable of affecting every major organ system in the body. Cortisol is also essential for the maintenance of normal organic and metabolic functions and participates in the stress response. Stress levels of cortisol activate the sympathetic nervous system to increase the release of stored glucose and fats and to suppress immune function. There are two forms of stress, short term (acute) and long term (chronic). For instance, a person may encounter acute stress when suddenly hearing a loud noise and chronic stress because of constant deadline pressure or having major difficulties with a spouse or family member. Michael Antoni (1993) and colleagues compiled the following symptoms of stress:

Cognitive symptoms: Feelings of anger, hostility, or difficulties with memory and concentration.

Emotional symptoms: Feelings of tension, irritability, restlessness, worries, inability to relax, sadness.

Behavioral symptoms: Avoidance of tasks; sleep problems; difficulty in completing work assignments; fidgeting; tremors; strained face; clenching fists; crying; changes in eating, drinking, or smoking behaviors.

Physiological symptoms: Tense or stiff muscles; grinding teeth; sweating; tension headaches; faint feelings; choking feeling; difficulty in swallowing; stomachache; nausea; vomiting; loosening of bowels; constipation; frequency and urgency of urination; loss of interest in sex; tiredness; shakiness or tremors; weight loss or gain; awareness of heartbeat.

Social symptoms: Some people under stress seek out others to be with, while others withdraw.

It is of vital importance to understand the physiology of stress to induce a positive parasympathetic state of relaxation to countervail the sympathetic responses. All stress management techniques aim to induce the parasympathetic state. Herbert Benson of the Harvard Medical School termed it the *relaxation response* (Goleman & Gurin, 1993). The traditional biomedical model has been effective in treating disease, but it has its shortcomings because it has no way to incorporate the knowledge that thoughts and emotions can enhance development of diseases or promote their cures.

This discussion leads into the next section on biopsychosocial models. The biopsychosocial models encompass the MindBody and spiritual domain in a person; therefore, they are reviewed in this chapter because health care practitioners are encouraged to make use of these models when assessing clients/patients.

BIOPSYCHOSOCIAL MODELS

To find new approaches to deal with burnout prevention, an effort has to be made to integrate and expand existing biopsychosocial models of health and disease. Key features and comparisons of (1) the traditional biomedical model, (2) the psychosocial model, (3) the human ecological system model, and (4) the psychoneuroimmunological (PNI) model are outlined and described.

Traditional Biomedical Model

Although effective at treating disease, the biomedical model has many shortcomings. In this model, the disease process and the treatment act on a passive organism, and the treatment and disease do not interact. Psychological processes such as the potential power of thoughts and emotions are left aside and not integrated in the biomedical model.

Psychosocial Model

The disease process interacts with the person, and psychological processes interact with physiological processes. The person interacts with the sociocultural environment. The treatment, the disease, and the environment are all capable of interacting as well. This model emphasizes the importance of seeing the disease and its treatment as an event that occurs, not as an isolated event at the cellular or organ level. In other words, one can begin to see that the physical aspects of the disease and the psychosocial and cultural processes are no longer clearly different. Thoughts and emotions are intimately connected to the workings of the human body (Lovallo, 1997). Constant job strain that manifests itself in physical, emotional, work-related, and interpersonal symptoms most often leads to burnout (Figley & Kleber, 1995). In terms of stress research as well as environmental and health action, the heuristic human ecological model is described next.

Psychoneuroimmunology

In recognition of the interactions among the nervous, endocrine, and immune systems and their bioregulatory implications, the exciting field of PNI, also called neuroimmunomodulation, neuroendocrine immunology, or behavioral neuroimmunology, has developed. These terms are all synonymous in the field of psychoneuroimmunology. However, the PNI term is widely mentioned in the literature, and is used by many health care practitioners. Stresses such as marital discord and caring for patients can produce changes in immune function of potential clinical importance; therefore, the PNI model is included in this literature review.

It is interesting to note that the PNI model has implications for the practice of medicine and nursing care (Solomon, 1997). First, to care for family members, the health care practitioner must take into account the family dynamics. Second, in the family context, gender as well as cultural and social perspectives are relevant to physical and mental well-being and to health-related behaviors such as smoking, drinking, and preventive activities. Third, as a consequence of the first two statements, the health care practitioner needs an understanding of the associations between disruption of immune function and any significant clinical consequences. Interventions such as stress reduction for health care practitioners themselves, their family members, and their patients may then be cost-effective in terms of days lost from work or acquired stress-related illness (Buckingham, Gillies, & Cowell, 1997).

Stress research tends to compare the environmental stimulus, the perception, and the effects on the body (e.g., immune response) with the effects on the body and its disease or recovery. Matalka and Sidki (1998) reported the effects of academic examination on cortisol and prolactin and total leukocyte, neutrophil, lymphocyte, and monocyte counts. This study found that examination stress significantly increased cortisol levels and circulating neutrophil counts. Prolactin levels also increased, but this finding was not significant. Cortisol is known to downregulate the immune system and the circulating leukocyte counts, which could compromise the immune system. It also inhibits production of interleukin 2 from T-helper cells and suppresses antigen presentation by macrophages. Academic stress increased cortisol level via ACTH release from the pituitary gland. This study could be useful for its application during the residency years, when residents encounter examination stress.

Cunningham (1981) outlined the work on psychological conditioning of immune responses as described by Ader as correlating levels between the ideas, expectations, and effects on the body. Described next is a model showing the levels through which an environmental stimulus, perceived by the mind, may affect events in the body and, eventually, health and behavior. It seems worthwhile to investigate whether white cell migration patterns can be altered by stress management techniques, such as meditation, biofeedback, visual imagery, and self-hypnosis, to mention a few. An understanding of the endocrine system sets the stage for the distinction between the inner (homeostasis) and the outer (adaptation). The integration of PNI with its nervous, neuroendocrine, and immune components sets the stage for a nonlinear, nonmechanistic understanding based on systems and informational theories. The body is more than a system of anatomy, physiology, and biochemistry or even psychosomatics and molecular biology. PNI is dissolving dualism of MindBody, body-environment, and individual-population. Levin and Solomon hypothesized that patients themselves will begin to understand their bodies in new ways. The degree to which the patient is skilled at sensing the body's stressors (precursors of diseases) and its health are also conditions of meaning as integrated through interpretations of life experienced by the mind-brain-immune system.

There is growing evidence for the extensive stress-related effects on neuroendocrine-immune interactions (Solomon, 1997). The *New England Journal of Medicine* published a report in 1991 showing a direct link between mental state and disease. That study demonstrated a striking correlation between levels of psychological stress and susceptibility to infection by a common cold virus. The researchers Ader and Cohen, in the mid-1970s found a number of physiological connections between the brain, the immune system, and stress-related illnesses. In sum, stress can suppress immune function, especially if someone has experienced a major disruption in life, such as a divorce, loss of a loved one, or a medical condition. Therefore, relaxation, group support, and other forms of stress management may well enhance immunity (Kiecolt-Glaser & Glaser, 1993).

MODELS OF FAMILY STRESS AND COPING

Stress and crisis are such common occurrences in the life of individuals and their partners that they seem to be a part of the human condition. Burnout is a process that emerges gradually. Not only is burnout a work-related concept, other environments or ecosystems play an important role in determining whether and to what degree a person will experience burnout. Burnout, a form of ecological dysfunction as viewed by (Carroll, 1980), means that a person, his or her ecosystems, and the reciprocal impact each has on the other must be understood. Personal signs of burnout as mentioned in this literature review should not only lead to strategies that correct that person's problem, but also should include an ecological system analysis that should prompt the development of a systemic intervention.

The following is a summary of some assumptions about burnout:

1. Burnout, a process, not an event, is caused by prolonged exposure to stress and frustration.
2. Various personal and environmental factors (stressors) that generate stress must be considered as potential causes of burnout.
3. Burnout is a holistic or biopsychosocial concept.
4. Burnout may occur in varying degrees, from loss of energy to a serious illness.
5. Burnout is not a disease, and the medical model is not an appropriate analytical model for understanding and coping with it.
6. Although certain characteristics are shared by all burned-out practitioners, burnout prevention efforts have to be individualized.
7. Burnout prevention programs have to focus on the person as the microsystem; the partner, spouse, and family as the mesosystem; the workplace and community as the exosystem; and the cultural/societal values and expectations as the macrosystem (Carroll & White, 1982). Although burnout as described by Carroll and White is not a disease, its emotional and physiological patterns could lead to disease. This author believes that self-management of emotions and cognition through stress-reducing methods might reduce stress and therefore not lead to burnout.

SUGGESTED READING

Borysenko, M. (1991). Psychoneuroimmunology: The interface between psychology and the immune system. In *In-Depth Perspectives On Psychoimmunology and the Mind/Body Connection. A Workbook.* The National Institute for the Clinical Application of Behavioral Medicine.

Buckingham, J. C., Gillies, G. E., & Cowell, A. (1997). *Stress, Stress Hormones and the Immune System.* New York: Wiley.

Carroll, J. F. X., & White, W. L. (1982). Theory building: Integrating individual and environmental factors within an ecological framework. In W. S. Paine (Ed.), *Job Stress and Burnout* (pp. 41–61). Beverly Hills, CA: Sage.

Cunningham, A. J. (1981). Mind, body and immune response. In R. Ader (Ed.). *Psychoneuroimmunology* (pp. 609–616). Orlando, FL: Academic Press.

Figley, C. R., & Kleber, R. J. (1995). Beyond the victim: Secondary traumatic stress. In R. J. Kleber, C. R. Figley, & P. R. Gerson (Eds.), *Beyond Trauma* (pp. 76–95). New York: Plenum Press.

Goleman, D., & Gurin, J. (1993). *Mind Body Medicine.* Yonkers, NY: Consumer Reports Books.

Ivancevich, J., & Matteson, M. (1981). Stress prevention framework for management. *Organizational Dynamics, 3,* 5–25.

Kiecolt-Glaser, J. K., & Glaser, R. (1993). Mind and immunity. In D. Goleman & J. Gurin (Eds.), *Mind Body Medicine* (pp. 19–39). Yonkers, NY: Consumer Reports Books.

Lovallo, W. R. (1997). *Stress and Health*. Thousand Oaks, CA: Sage.

Maslach, C. (1976). *Burnout: A social psychological analysis*. Unpublished manuscript, University of California, Berkeley.

Matalka, K. Z., & Sidki, A. (1998). Academic stress—influence on leukocyte distribution, cortisol, and prolactin. *Laboratory Medicine, 29*, 697–702.

Plaut, S. M., & Friedman, S. M. (1981). Psychosocial factors in infectious disease. In R. Ader (Ed.), *Psychoneuroimmunology* (pp. 3–26). Orlando, FL: Academic Press.

Schafer, W. (1996). *Stress Management for Wellness*. Orlando, FL: Holt, Rinehart & Winston.

Selye, H. (1980). *Seyle's Guide to Stress Research*. New York: Van Nostrand Reinhold.

Solomon, F. G. (1997). Clinical and social implications of stress-induced neuroendocrine-immune interactions. In J. C. Buckingham, G. E. Gillies, & A. M. Cowell (Eds.), *Stress, Stress Hormones and the Immune System* (pp. 385–401). New York: Wiley.

Appendix D

Further Thoughts on the Topic of Energy and Its Role in MindBody Medicine

There are three major aspects of energy systems: chakras, auras (the biofield), and meridians.

CHAKRAS

There are seven major *chakras* (energy centers), and clients can learn how to reduce anxiety and enhance a sense of vitality in each center. Interestingly, the chakra sequence presents itself also in Maslow's hierarchy of needs. According to Maslow, there are seven levels of needs; however, most likely you were taught only the five needs of Maslow's hierarchy (Slater, 2000, p.132). Here is a review of Maslow's pyramid: physiologic-survival needs; need for safety; need for love and belonging; need for esteem; need for self-actualization; need to know and understand; and aesthetic needs (Dossey, Keegan, & Guzzetta, 2000).

Chakras are associated with major nerve plexi and with the pituitary and pineal neuroendocrine glands. Chakras are assigned the colors of the rainbow and the tones of an octave. The researcher Hiroshi Motoyama of Japan found that "subjects who could consciously project energy through their Chakras displayed significant electrical field disturbance over the activated Chakras" (Slater, 2000, pp. 136–137). Another researcher, Hunt Valerie at the University of California at Los Angeles, placed electromyographic electrodes on the skin of chakra areas and found regular, high-frequency, wavelike electrical signals from 100 to 1,600 cycles per second. For example, the frequency band of brain waves is between 1 and 100 cycles per second. It is of great importance to understand that it is the individual's decision to heal and not the expertise of the health care professional. Every person has a choice of making use of the mental activities for his or her own healing system. Motoyama's research findings suggest that people can consciously project energy through their chakras and control their own energy (Dossey, Keegan, & Guzzetta, 2000, p. 136-137).

MERIDIANS

The meridian system in the body transports energy in a way an artery transports blood to adjust the metabolism and the cellular change in our bodies. *Meridians* are life forces and affect every physiological system, including the immune and lymphatic systems. If a meridian is obstructed, then the system is out of balance. In Chinese tradition, there are 12 pairs of meridians that carry human energy, called *chi* by the Chinese and *qi* by the Japanese. Along the meridian pathways, there are acupuncture points that can be stimulated by pressure, needles, or temperature. Meridians carry the names of the organs; however, they are not always equated with the organ of their name because the Chinese tradition prohibits autopsies. Chinese tradition mostly relied on observations of the meridian's function. For example, the kidney meridian refers to the area of influence of that meridian, not the organ by the same name. Radioactive studies also suggest that the meridian system is separate from the vascular and lymphatic system.

Acupressure and acupuncture techniques work directly with meridians to bring organs into balance. It is hypothesized that any meridian technique is either to calm a hyperalert meridian system or to stimulate a sluggish one (Dossey et al., (2000). Meridian-based therapies use pressure points along acupuncture meridians to release negative patterns of emotional and physical response. Examples of such therapies are thought field therapy, the emotional freedom technique, the Tapas acupressure technique, and other variations of these approaches. One of the great advantages of these techniques is that clients can be taught to use any of those techniques on their own as self-healing. According to the literature, no side effects have been reported by using those techniques. Clients who experience post-traumatic stress, anxiety, poor self-esteem, and phobias are helped by these therapies (Benor, 2002).

AURAS

The *aura*, an atmosphere or luminous glow surrounding something, is complemented by the meridians and by the chakras. Brennan describes the aura as a seven-layer system. It includes the physical, astral, and spiritual planes. The structured layers appear to be standing waves of light patterns with small electrical charges moving along them. The layers are interpenetrating and constantly moving all the other layers, including the physical body. Interestingly, each layer is associated with a chakra. Kunz described the aura as dense light and as "the personal emotional field." Brennan's description of the aura as layers of magnetic density that surround a physical body and diminish in intensity as one moves further away from subtle energy systems in their body and to influence their healing and to improve their health body resembles a physic's descriptions of an electromagnetic field (Dossey et al., 2000).

The research study Active Ingredient Project directed by Figley and Carbonell (1995) at Florida State University in 1995 looked at the most effective method for relief of post-traumatic stress as compared with other treatment/therapy modalities such as Eye Movement Reprocessing and Desensitization (EMDR). The researchers studied and worked with the meridians and their specific acupoints to relieve emotional stress. The tapping of specific acupressure points along 14 major meridians showed clinical relief of generalized anxiety, fears, and worry as well as phobia and post-traumatic stress. Psychologists Callahan (1996) and Gallo (1998) successfully studied specific acupoints, also called algorithms as described in Gallo (1999).

SUGGESTED READING

Benor, D.J. (2000). Intuitive diagnostics. In Dossey, B.M., Keegan, L., & Guzzetta, C.E. (2000). *Holistic Nursing.* Gaithersburg, MD: Aspen.

Dossey, B.M., Keegan, L., & Guzzetta, C.E. (2000). *Holistic Nursing.* Gaithersburg, MD: Aspen.

Slater, V.E. (2000). Energetic healing. In Dossey, B.M., Keegan, L., & Guzzetta, C.E. (Eds.). *Holistic Nursing.* Gaithersburg, MD: Aspen.

Bibliography

Academy of Science. *Proceedings of the National Academy of Science.* Retrieved November 30, 2004, from the academy Web site, www.nasonline.org.

Achterberg, J., Dossey, B., & Kolkmeier, L. (1994). *Rituals of Healing.* New York: Bantam Books.

Achterberg, J., & Rider, M.S. (1993). The effects of music mediated imagery on neutrophils and lymphocytes. *Biofeedback and Self Regulation, 14,* 247–257.

Ader, R. (1990). *Psychoneuroimmunology.* San Diego: Academic Press.

Alexander, D., Monk, J.S., & Jonas, A.P. (1985). Occupational stress, personal strain, and coping among residents and faculty members. *Journal of Medical Education, 60.*

Allison, N. (Ed.). (1999). *The Complete Body, Mind, and Spirit.* Chicago: Keats.

Altenmueller, E.O. (2005). Music in your head. *Scientific American Mind,* Special Edition, 24–31.

American Academy of Family Physicians. (1998). *Facts About Family Practice.* Kansas City, MO: American Academy of Family Physicians.

Antoni, M.H. (1993). Stress management: Strategies that work. In D. Goleman & J. Gurin (Eds.), *Mind Body Medicine* (pp. 385–401). Yonkers, NY: Consumer Reports Books.

Antonie, M. (1995). Stress management intervention. Cited in *Monitor of the American Psychological Association.*

Antonuccio, D.O., Thomas, M. & Danton, W.G. (1997). A cost-effectiveness analysis of cognitive behavior therapy and fluoxetine (Prozac) in the treatment of depression. *Behavior Therapy,* 28, 187-210.

Arnetz, B.B. (1991). White collar stress: What studies of physicians can teach us. *Psychotherapy Psychosomatic, 55,* 197–200.

Ashford, J.B., LeCroy, C.W., & Lortie, K.L. (2006). *Human Behavior in the Social Environment.* Belmont, CA: Thomson Brooks/Cole.

Astin, J. (2000). The efficacy of distant healing: A systematic review of randomized trials. *American Intern. Med., 132,* 903–910.

Astin, J., et al. (2003). Mind-Body medicine. State of the science, implication for practice. *Journal of the American Board of Family Practice, 16,* 131–147.

Barabasz, M. (1989). Treatment of bulimia with hypnosis involving awareness and control in clients with high dissociative capacity. *International Journal* of *Psychosomatic Medicine, 36,* 104–108.

Barabasz, M., & Spiegel, D. (1989). Hypnotizability and weight loss in obese subjects. *International Journal of Eating Disorders, 8,* 335–341.

Barlow, D. (2000). Cognitive behavioral therapy, imipramine or their combination for panic disorders: A randomized controlled trial. *Journal of the American Medical Association, 283,* 2529–2536.

Barlow, D.H. (1996). Advances in psychosocial treatment of anxiety disorders. *Archives of General Psychiatry, 53*, 727–735.

Barnes, V. (1999). Acute effects of transcendental meditation on hemodynamic functioning in middle age adults. *Psychosomatic Medicine, 61*(4), 525-531.

Barnes, V. (2003). Impact of transcendental meditation on cardiovascular function at rest and during acute stress in adolescents with high normal blood pressure. *Journal of Psychosomatic Research, 51*, 597–605.

Beck, A.T., & Tan, S. (1996). Report on psychoneuroimmunology. *Research Society Meeting.*

Bennet, H. (1986). Behavioral anesthesia. *Advances, 2.*

Bennet, H., & Benan, D.R. (1985). *Journal of Anesthesiology.*

Bennett, M.P., & Lengacher, C.A. (2006). Humor and laughter may influence health. I. History and background. *Evidence-Based Complementary and Alternative Medicine, 3*, 61–63.

Bennett, M.P., Zeller, J.M., Rosenberg, L., & McCann, J. (2003). The effects of mindful laughter on stress and natural killer cell activity. *Alternative Therapies in Health and Medicine, 9*, 92) 38–45.

Benor, D.J. (2002). Energy medicine for the internist. *Medical Clinics of North America, 86.*

Black, P.H. (1994). Psychoneuroendocrinology of stress and its immune consequences, *Antimicrob Agents Chemotherapy, 38*, 1–6.

Blanchard, E., & Malamood, H.S (1996). Psychological treatment of irritable bowel syndrome. *Professional Psychology: Research and Practice, 27*, 241-244.

Blanchard, E.B., & Scharff, L. (2002). Psychosocial aspects of assessment and treatment of irritable bowel syndrome in adults and recurrent abdominal pain in children. *Journal of Consulting and Clinical Psychology, 70*, 725–738.

Blumental, J.A., et al. (1997). Stress management and exercise training cardiac patients with myocardial ischemia. *Archives of Internal Medicine*, 157, 2213–2223.

Borysenko, M. (1991). Psychoneuroimmunology: The interface between psychology and the immune system. The National Institute for the Clinical Application of Behavioral Medicine. *In-Depth Perspectives on Psychoimmunology and the Mind/Body Connection, a Workbook.*

Bosnak, K. (2002, May 2–4). *Use of dreams for physical health.* Report presented at Harvard's program in science and MindBody medicine, Cambridge, MA.

Breznitz, S., & Goldberger, L. (1993). *Stress Research at a Crossroads.* New York: Free Press.

Brigham, D.D. (1990). *The Use of Imagery in a Multimodal Psycho-neuro-immunology Program for Cancer and Other Chronic Diseases.* New York: Plenum Press.

Broadbent, E., Petrie, K.J., Alley, P.G., & Booth, R.J. (2003). Psychological stress impairs early wound repair following surgery. *Psychosomatic Medicine, 65*, 865–869.

Brosschot, J.F., et al. (1994). Influence of life stress on immunological reactivity to mild psychological stress. *Psychosomatic Medicine, 56*, 216–224.

Brown. (2003). *Journal of Personal and Social Psychology.*

Brown, B., Werner, C.M., & Kim, N. (2003). Personal and contextual supports to change. *Journal of Personality and Social Psychology, 41*, 1094–1104.

Brown, G. (2005). Cognitive therapy reduces suicide risk. *Journal of the American Medical Association, 294*, 563–70, 623–624.

Brown, K.W. (2003). The benefits of being present: Mindfulness and its role in psychological well-being. *Journal of Personal and Social Psychology, 84*, 822–848.

Buckingham, J.C., Gillies, G.E., & Cowell, A. (1997*). Stress, Stress Hormones and the Immune System.* New York: Wiley.

Byrd, R.C. (1988). Positive therapeutic effects of intercessory prayer in a coronary care unit population. *Southern Medical Journal, 18* (7), 826–829.

Cadigan, M.E., Caruao, N.A., Halderman, S.M., et al. (2001) The effects of music on cardiac patients on bed rest. *Progress in Cardiovascular Nursing, 16*, 5–13.

Cain, E.N., et al. (1986). Psychosocial benefits of a cancer support group. *Cancer, 57*, 183–189.

Calvert, E.L., Houghton, L.A., Cooper, P., Morris, J., & Whorwell, P.J. (2002). Long-term improvement in functional dyspepsia using hypnotherapy. *Gastroenterology, 123*, 1778–1785.

Canino, E., Cordona, R., et al. (1994). A behavioral treatment program as a therapy in the control of primary hypertension. *Acta Cientific Venezolana, 45*, 23–30.

Carpenter, A. (1998). *Kant's earliest solution to the mind/body problem.* Unpublished doctoral dissertation, University of California at Berkley. Retrieved from: http://www.andrewcarpenter.net/diss/diss_pdf_.html.

Carroll, J.F.X., & White, W.L. (1982). Theory building: Integrating individual and environmental factors within an ecological framework. In W. S. Paine (Ed.), *Job Stress and Burnout* (pp. 41–61). Beverly Hills, CA: Sage.

Castes, M., Hagel, I., et al. (1999) Immunologic changes associated with clinical improvement of asthmatic children subjected to psychosocial intervention. *Brain, Behavior and Immunity, 13*, 1–13.

Castillo-Richmond, A. & Schneider, R.H. (2002). Effects of stress reduction on carotid atherosclerosis in hypertensive African Americans. *Stroke, 31*, 568.

Caudill, M., et al. (1991). Decreased use by chronic pain patients: Response to behavioral medicine interventions. *Journal of Chronic Pain, 7*, 305.–310.

Cha, K.Y., Wirth, D.P., & Lobo, R.A. (2001). Does prayer influence the success of in vitro fertilization-embryo transfer? Report of a masked, randomized trial. *Journal of Reproductive Medicine, 46*, 781–787.

Chamberlin, J. (2006). A picture of health: A psychologist's multidimensional employee wellness initiative at the University of Missouri emphasizes mind-body health. *Monitor on Psychology, 57*, 30–31.

Chang, P. (2002). Angry personality increases heart attack risks fivefold. *Archives of Internal Medicine, 162*, 901–906.

Chen, E.J.M. (2000). Behavioral and cognitive interventions in the treatment of pain in children. *Pediatric Clinics of North America, 47.*

Classen, C., et al. (2001). Supportive-expressive group therapy and distress in patients with metastatic breast cancer. A randomized clinical intervention trial. *Archive of General Psychiatry, 58*, 494–501.

Cohen, S. (1997). Psychosocial stress and susceptibility to the common cold. *New England Journal of Medicine, 325*, 606–612.

Cohen, S., Doyle, W., Turner, R.B., et al. (2003). Emotional style and susceptivity to the common cold. *Psychosomatic Medicine, 65*, 652–657.

Cohen, S.O., & Walco, G.A. (1999). Dance/movement therapy for children and adolescents with cancer. *Cancer Practice, 7*, 34–42.

Cohen, F., Kemeny, M.E., Kearney, K.A., Zegans, L.S., Neuhaus, J.M., & Conant, M.A. (1999). Persistent stress as a predictor of genital herpes recurrence. *Archives of Internal Medicine, 159* (20), 2430–2436.

Cole, S. (2003). Social identity and physical health. *Journal of Personal and Social Psychology*, 72, 320–336.

Connolly, K. (2004). *Brain activity and the development of posttraumatic stress disorder.* Unpublished research paper, Florida State University, College of Social Work.

Cousins, N. (1990). *Head First: The Biology of Hope and the Healing Power of the Human Spirit.* New York: Viking Penguin.

Cowles, L.A.F. (2004). *Social Work in the Health Field: A Case Perspective.* Binghamton, NY: Haworth Press.

Crane, D.R. (1997). Why marital therapy matters: The economic and social consequences of divorce. In *Fundamentals of Marital Therapy.* New York: Brunner/Mazel.

Cruess, D.G. (2000). *Psychosomatic Medicine, 62,* 304–308.

Cunningham, A.J. (1981). Mind, body and immune response. In R. Ader (Ed.). *Psychoneuroimmunology* (pp. 609–616). Orlando, FL: Academic Press.

Cunningham, A.J., Phillips, C., Lockwood, G.A., Hedley, D.W., & Edmonds, C.V.I. (2000). Association of involvement in psychological self-regulation with longer survival in patients with metastatic cancer: An exploratory study. *Advances in Mind-Body Medicine, 16,* 176–294.

Cunningham, A. J., & Tocco, E.K. (1989). A randomized trial of group psychoeducational therapy for cancer patients. *Patient Education and Counseling, 14,* 101–114.

Davidson, K., et al. (2002). Constructive venting behavior predicts blood pressure in a population based sample. *Health Psychology, 19,* 55–64.

Davidson, K., et al. (2003). Evidence-based behavioral medicine: What is it and how do we achieve it? *Annals of Behavioral Medicine, 26,* 161–171.

Davidson, R.J., et al. (2003). Alterations in brain and immune function produced by mindfulness meditation. *Psychosomatic Medicine, 65,* 564–570.

Davis, D. (2002, November 9–10). *Guided imagery prepares patients for surgery while reducing charges for care: A health plan sponsored program.* Report from Blue Shield of California presented at the Society of Clinical and Experimental Hypnosis 53rd annual scientific program, Boston.

Dean, C. (1989). Do psychosocial factors predict survival? *Journal of Psychosomatic Research, 33,* 561–569.

Dean, R.A., & Gregory, D.M. (2005). More than trivial: Strategies for using palliative care. *Cancer Nursing, 28,* 292–300.

Del Pozo, J.M., et al. (2004). Biofeedback treatment increases heart rate variability in patients with known coronary artery disease. *American Heart Journal, 147,* E11.

Derogatis, L.R., Abeloff, M.D., & Melisaratos, N. (1979). Psychological coping mechanisms and survival time in metastatic breast cancer. *Journal of American Medical Association, 242,* 1504–1508.

Dienstfrey, H. (1996). One view of 14 responses to five questions. *Advances 12* (3), 37.

Dittmann, M. (2003). Coping with cancer through social connection. *Monitor on Psychology,* 24–26.

Dolaba, K., & Fox, C. (1999). The effects of guided imagery on comfort of women with early stage breast cancer undergoing radiation therapy. *Oncology Nursing Forum, 26,* 67–72.

Dossey, B.M., Keegan, L., & Guzzetta, C.E. (2000). *Holistic Nursing.* Gaithersburg, MD: Aspen.

Dossey, L. (1993). *Healing Words: The Power of Prayer and the Practice of Medicine.* San Francisco: Harper Collins.

Dossey, L. (1999). *Reinventing Medicine: Beyond Mind Body to a New Area of Healing.* San Francisco: Harper.

Doyle, Cohen, et al. (2003). Emotional style and susceptibility to the common cold. *Psychosomatic Medicine, 65,* 652–657.

Dreher, H. (1993). Mind-Body research and its detractors. *Advances, 9,* 59–62.

Dreher, H. (1998). Mind-Body interventions for surgery: Evidence and exigency. *Advances, 14,* 207–222.

Dreher, H. (2001). A challenge to the mind-body health movement. *Advances in Mind-Body Medicine, 17,* 147–150.

Drossman, D.A. (2000). AGA technical review on irritable bowel syndrome. *Gastroenterology,* 123, 2108–2131

Enck, P. (1992). Biofeedback training in disordered defecation. *Digestive Disease, 38,* 1953–1960.

Eng, P.M., Fitzmaurice, et al. (2003). Anger expression and risk of coronary artery disease among male health professionals. *Psychosomatic Medicine, 65,* 100–110.

Epstein, G. (1996). Mind-body medicine and biological medicine: An unbridgeable gap. *Advances: Journal of Mind Body Health, 12* (3).

Esch, T., Stefano, G., Fricchione, G., & Benson, H. (2002). Stress in cardiovascular disease. *Medical Science Monitor, 8,* RA93–RA101.

Esplen, M.J., et al. (1998). A randomized controlled trial of guided imagery in bulimia nervosa. *Psychological Medicine, 28,* 1347–1357.

Everson, S.A., et al. (1996). Hopelessness and risk of mortality and incident of myocardial infarction and cancer. *Psychosomatic Medicine, 58,* 113–121.

Fava, G., Grandi, S., Zielezny, M., et al. (1994). Cognitive behavioral treatment of residual symptoms in primary major depressive disorder. *American Journal of Psychiatry, 151,* 1295–1299.

Fawzy, F.I. (1995). Critical review of psychosocial intervention and cancer care. *Archives of General Psychiatry, 52,* 100–1300.

Fawzy, F.I., et al. (1993). Malignant melanoma: Effects of an early structured psychiatric intervention. *Archives of General Psychiatry, 50,* 681–689.

Fawzy, F.I. (1995). Critical review of psychosocial intervention and cancer care. *Archives of General Psychiatry, 52,* 100–1300.

Fawzy & Fawzy. (1993). Malignant melanoma. *Archives of General Psychiatry, 50,* 681–689.

Figley, C.R., & Carbonell, J.L. (1995). Active ingredients project: The systematic clinical demonstration of the most efficient treatments of PTSD. In F. P. Gallo (Ed.), *Energy Psychology* (p. 25). New York: CRC Press.

Figley, C. (1995). *Compassion Fatigue.* New York: Brunner/Mazel.

Figley, C. (1998). *Burnout in Families.* Boca Raton, FL: CRC Press.

Figley, C. R., & Kleber, R.J. (1995). Beyond the victim: Secondary traumatic stress. In R.J. Kleber, C.R. Figley, & P.R. Gersons (Eds.), *Beyond Trauma* (pp. 76–95). New York: Plenum Press.

Fry, W. (1992). The physiological effects of humor, mirth, and laughter. *Journal of the American Medical Association, 267,* 1857–1858.

Gallo, F. (1998). *Energy Psychology.* Boca Raton, FL: CRC Press.

Gallo, F. (1999). *Innovations in Psychology.* Boca Raton, FL: CRC Press.

Gallo, L. (1999). *Energy Medicine, 61* (4).

Galper, D.I., Taylor, A.G., & Cox, D.J. (2003). Current status of mind-body intervention for vascular complication of diabetes. *Family Community Health, 26,* 34–40.

Gaynor, L.M. (2000). *Sounds of healing: A physician reveals the therapeutic power of sound, voice, and music.* Broadway Books.

Glassman, A.H., & Shapiro, P.A. (1998). Depression and the course of coronary artery disease. *American Journal of Psychiatry, 155,* 4–11.

Garfinkel, M.S., Singhal, A., Katz, W.A., et al. (1998). Yoga-based intervention for carpal tunnel syndrome: A randomized controlled trial. *Journal of the American Medical Association, 280*(18), 1601–1603.

Goleman, D., & Gurin, J. (1993). *Mind Body Medicine.* Yonkers, NY: Consumer Reports Books.

Gonsalkorale, W.M., Houghton, L.A., & Whorwell, P.J. (2002). Hypnotherapy in irritable bowel syndrome: A large-scale audit of a clinical service with examination of factors influencing responsiveness. *American Journal of Gastroenterology, 97,* 954–961.

Good, M., Anderson, G.C., Stanton-Hicks, M., et al. (2002) Relaxation and music reduce pain after gynecologic surgery. *Pain Management Nursing, 3,* 61–70.

Goodman, M. (1994). An hypothesis explaining the successful treatment of psoriasis. *Thermal Biofeedback and Self-Regulation, 19,* 347–352.

Greer, P. (2001). Breast cancer: Imaginal realms of meaning. *Journal of Poetry Therapy, 14.*

Greer, S. (2000). Psychological response to breast cancer. *Lancet, 49.*

Grossbart, T. (1993). The skin matters of the flesh. In D. Goleman (Ed.), *Mind Body Medicine* (pp 145-175). Yonkers, NY: Consumer Reports Books.

Grzywacz, J.C. (2004). Toward health promotion: Physical and social behavior in complete health. *American Journal of Health Behavior, 28,* 99–111.

Guillemont, F., et al. (1994). Biofeedback for the treatment of fecal incontinence. *Diseases of the Colon and Rectum, 38,* 393–397.

Gump, B., et al. (2004). Depressive symptoms and mortality in men: Results from the Multiple Risk Factor Interventions Trial. *Stroke, 36,* 98–102.

Guyton, A. (1991). *Textbook of Medical Physiology.* New York: Saunders.

Guzzetta, C. (1989). Effects of relaxation and music therapy on patients in a coronary care unit with presumptive acute myocardial infarction. *Heart Lung, 18,* 609–616.

Hafen, B.Q., Karren, K.J., Frandsen, K.J., & Smith, N.L. (1996). *Mind Body Health.* Needham Heights, MA: Simon & Schuster.

Harris, W.S., Harris, W.S., Gowda, M., Kolb, J.W., Strychacz, C.P., Vacek, J.L., Jones, P.G., Forker, A., O'Keefe, J.H., & McCalliste (1999). A randomized, controlled trial of the effects of remote, intercessory prayer on outcomes in patients admitted to the coronary care unit. *Archive Internal Medicine, 159,* 2273–2278.

Hart, E. (1995). *Creative Loop: How the Brain Makes a Mind.* New York: Addison-Wesley.

Harvey, R.T., Hinton, R.A., Gunary, R.M., & Barry, R.E. (1989). Individual and group hypnotherapy in treatment of refractory irritable bowel syndrome. *Lancet, 8635,* 424–425.

Kabat-Zinn, J. (1986). Four-year follow up of a meditation based program for the self-regulation of chronic pain. *Clinical Journal of Pain 2,* 150–173.

Haymamm-Monnikes, A.R., Flound, & Kabat-Zinn, J. (1986). Four-year follow up of a meditation based program for the self-regulation of chronic pain. *Clinical Journal of Pain 2*, 150–173.

Haymamm-Monnikes, A.R., Flound, & Kabat-Zinn, J. (2000). The combination of medical treatment plus multi-component behavioral therapy is superior to medical treatment alone in the therapy of irritable bowel syndrome. *American Journal of Gastroenterology, 95*, 944–981.

Hellman, C.J., et al. (1990). The study of the effectiveness of two group behavioral medicine interventions for patients with psychosomatic complaints. *Behavioral Medicine, 16*, 165–175.

Herron, R.E., Hills, S.L., et al. (1996). The impact of the transcendental meditation program on government payments to physicians in Quebec. *American Journal of Health Promotion, 10*, 208–216.

Heymen, S., Wexner, S.D., Vickers, D., Nogueras, J.J., Weiss, E.G., & Pikarsky, A.L. (1999). Prospective randomized trial comparing four biofeedback techniques for patients with constipation. *Diseases of the Colon and Rectum, 42*, 1388–1393.

Hinrichs, B. (1998). Computing the mind: A scientific approach to the philosophy of mind and brain. *The Humanist, 58*, 28–30.

Hiratsuka, J. (1990). Brief mental health care can reduce medical bill, four-year study confirms. *NASW News, 35.*

Hodges, C., Castro, C, Messer, S. (2004). Combat duty in Iraq and Afghanistan, mental health problem and barriers to cure. *New England Journal of Medicine, 351*, 13–22.

Holiday, S. (2002). Have fun while you can, you are only as old as you feel, don't even get old. An examination of memorable messages about aging. *Journal of Communication, 52*, 681–697.

Hover-Kramer, D. (1999). Comprehensive energy psychology: Emerging concepts for integrative psychologists. *San Diego Psychologist, 8*(5).

Hunter, M.S., & Liao, K.L.M. (March 1995). *Evaluation of a four session cognitive behavioral intervention for menopausal hot flashes.* Paper presented at British Psychological Society annual conference.

Hymann, M. (2000); *American Journal of Gastroenterology*; 95(4), 981–999.

Irwin, M. (1992). Depression: Central corticotropic releasing factor activates the autonomic nervous system and reduces natural killer cell activity. In N. Schneiderman et al. (Eds.), *Stress and Disease Process.* Mahwah, NJ: Erlbaum.

Ivancevich, J., & Matteson, M. (1981). Stress prevention framework for management. *Organizational Dynamics, 3*, 5–25.

Jacob, G.D. (2004). Cognitive behavior therapy and pharmacotherapy for insomnia: A randomized control trial and direct comparison. *Archives of Internal Medicine, 164*, 1888–1896.

Kabat-Zinn, J. (1986). Four-year follow up of a meditation based program for the self-regulation of chronic pain. *Clinical Journal of Pain 2*, 150–173.

Kabat-Zinn, J. (2000). Report of the annual Harvard Scientific Conference on Alternative Medicine. *Psychosomatic Medicine*, (1998) *60*, 625–632.

Kabat-Zinn, J., et al. (1992). Effectiveness of a meditation based stress reduction program in the treatment of anxiety disorders. *American Journal of Psychology, 149*, 936–994.

Kabat-Zinn, J., et al. (1998). Influence of a mindfulness meditation-based stress reduction intervention on rates of skin clearing in patients with moderate to severe psoriasis undergoing phototherapy and photochemotherapy. *Psychosomatic Medicine, 60*, 625–632.

Kant, I. (1998). Critique of Pure Reason (P. Guyer, Trans.). In P. Guyer and A. W. Wood (Eds.), *The Cambridge Edition of the Works of Immanuel Kant*. Cambridge, UK: Cambridge University Press.

Keller, E. (1993). *The effects of therapeutic touch on tension headache pain*. Master's thesis, University of Missouri, Columbia.

Keller, M.B. (2000). A comparison of nefrazodone, cognitive behavioral analysis system of psychotherapy, and their combination in the treatment of chronic depression. *New England Journal of Medicine, 342:* 1462–1470.

Kennell, J., Klaus, M., McGrath, S., Robertson, S., & Hinkley, C. (1992). Psychological support during childbirth. *Jordemodern, 105*(9), 308–310.

Kenney, J.W. (2000). Women's "inner-balance": A comparison of stressors, personality traits and health problems by age groups. *Journal of Advanced Nursing, 31*, 639–650.

Kiecolt-Glaser, J.K., Glaser, R., Williger, D., Stout, J., Messick. (1985). Psycho-social enhancement of immunocompetence in a geriatric population. *Health Psychology, 4*, 25–29.

Kiecolt-Glaser, J.K., & Glaser, R. (1993). Mind and immunity. In D. Goleman & J. Gurin (Eds.), *Mind Body Medicine* (pp. 19–39). Yonkers, NY: Consumer Reports Books.

Kiecolt-Glaser, J.K., et al. (1995). Slowing of wound healing by psychological stress. *Lancet, 346*, 1194–1196.

Kiecolt-Glaser, J.K., et al. (1998). Marital stress: Immunologic, neuroendocrine, and autonomic correlates. *Annals of the New York Academy of Science, 840*, 656–666.

Kivimaki, M., Leino-Arjas, P., et al. (2002). Work stress and risk of cardiovascular mortality. Prospective cohort study of industrial employees. *British Medical Journal, 19*, 7369–857.

Kivimaki, M., Leino-Arjas, P., et al. (2004). Work stress and incidence of newly diagnosed fibromalagia: perspective cohort study, *Journal of Psychonotic Research, 57*, 417–422.

Knight, W.E. (2002). Relaxing music prevents stress-induced increases in subjective anxiety, systolic blood pressure, and heart rate in healthy males and females. *Journal of Music Therapy, 38*, 254–272.

Kugelman, R. (1992). *Stress: The Nature and History of Engineered Grief.* Westport, CT: Praeger.

Kuhn, D. (2002). The effects of active and passive participation in musical activity on the immune system as measured by salivary immunoglobulin. *Journal of Music Therapy, 39*, 30–39.

Kwekkenboom, K. et al. (1998). Imaging ability and effective use of guided imagery. *Research in Nurse Health, 21*, 189–198.

Lang, D.V., Berotsh, E.G., & Fick, L.J. (2000). Adjunctive non-pharmacological analgesia for medical procedures. *Lancet, 355*, 1486–1490.

Lapore, S.J. (1997). Expressive writing moderates the relation between intrusive thoughts and depressive symptoms. *Journal of Personality and Social Psychology, 73*, 1030–1039.

LaPuma. (1999). Writing therapy to reduce asthma and RA symptoms. *Alternative Medicine Alert,* 2, 82–83.

Lawler, K.A., Younger, J.W., Piferi, R.L., Billington, E., Jobe, R, Edmondson, K. et al. (2003). A change of heart: Cardiovascular correlates of forgiveness in response to interpersonal conflict. *Journal of Behavior Medicine, 26,* 373–393.

Lehrer, P.M., (March 23, 1998). Emotionally triggered asthma: a review of research literature and some hypotheses for self regulation therapies. *Application Psychophysical Biofeedback,* 13–41.

Lepore, S.J. (1997). Expressive writing moderates the relation between intrusive thoughts and depressive symptoms. *Journal of Personality and Social Psychology, 73,* 1030–1037.

Lerner, M. (2000). Mind-body health at 25: An assessment. *Advances in Mind-Body Medicine, 16,* 295.

Lesperance, F., & Fansure-Smith, N. (2000). Depression in patients with cardiac disease. A practical review. *Journal of Psychosomatic Research, 48,* 379–391.

Level, M. (1994). *Archives of Family Medicine, 3,* 881–887.

Levin, J.S., Wickramasekera, I. E., & Hirshberg, C. (1998). *Is Religiousness a Correlate of Absorption? Implications for Psychophysiology, Coping, and Morbidity.* Rockville, MD: National Institute for Healthcare Research.

Linden, W.C. (1994). Clinical effectiveness of non-drug treatment for hypertension. A meta-analysis. *Annuals of Behavioral Medicine, 16,* 35–45.

Liossi, C., & Hatura, P. (2003). Clinical hypnosis in the alleviation of procedure related pain in pediatric oncology patients. *International Journal of Clinical and Experiential Hypnosis, 57.*

Lorig, K.R., Mazonso, P.D., Holman, H.R., & Mazonson. (1993). Evidence suggesting that health education for self management in patients with chronic arthritis has sustained health benefits while reducing health care costs. *Arthritis and Rheumatoid Arthritis, 36,* 439–446.

Lovallo, W.R. (1997). *Stress and Health.* Thousand Oaks, CA: Sage.

Lloyd, A.J. (2004). A toolbox for humanity: More than 9000 years of thought. *The Great Books of the Western World.* Encyclopedia Britannica.

Lutgendorf, S.K., Michael, H.A., Gail, I., Klimas, N., Fletcher, M.N., & Schneiderman, N. (1997). Cognitive processing style, mood, and immune function following HIV seropositivity notification. *Cognitive Therapy and Research, 21* (2), 157–184.

Lyketsos, C., et. al (1993). Depressive symptoms as predictors of medical outcomes in HIV infection. *Journal of the American Medical Association, 270,* 2563–2567.

Malchiodi, C. (2001). Art therapy. In N. Allison (Ed.). *The Complete Body, Mind, and Spirit* (pp. 311–312). New York: McGraw-Hill.

Mannion, M. (1997). Wilhelm Reich, 1897–1957. *Alternative and Complementary Therapies,* 3, 194.

Marcus, J., Elkins, G., & Mott, F. (2003). The integration of hypnosis into a model of palliative care. *Integrative Cancer Therapy, 2,* 365–370.

Martelli, M. F., et al. (2004). Psychological, neurological and medical consultation, assessment and management of pain. *Journal of Head Trauma Rehabilitation, 19,* 10–18.

Maslach, C. (1976). *Burnout: A social psychological analysis.* Unpublished manuscript, University of California, Berkeley.

Matalka, K.Z., & Sidki, A. (1998). Academic stress—influence on leukocyte distribution, cortisol, and prolactin. *Laboratory Medicine, 29,* 697–702.

Matheson, G.D. (1990). Psychological preparation of the patient for breast reconstruction. *Annals of Plastic Surgery, 24,* 238–247.

Matthews, D.A., Marlowe, S.M., & MacNutt, F.S. (2000). Effects of intercessory prayer on patients with rheumatoid arthritis. *Southern Medical Journal, 93*(12), 1177–1186.

Mazonson, L., et al. (1993). Evidence suggesting that health education for self management in patients with chronic arthritis has sustained health benefits while reducing health care cost. *Arthritis and Rheumatism, 36,* 439–446.

Mazza, N. (2001). The place of the poetic in dealing with death and loss. *Journal of Poetry Therapy, 15,* 29–35.

Mazza, N. (2003) Editor's note: The foundation and future of scholarship in poetry therapy. *Journal of Poetry Therapy, 16,* 1–4.

McDowell, B.J., et al. (1999). Effectiveness of behavioral therapy to treat incontinence in homebound older adults. *Journal of the American Geriatrics Society, 47,* 309–318.

McEwen. B.S. (1993). Stress and the individual mechanisms leading to disease. *Archives of Internal Medicine, 153,* 2093–2101.

McMahon, K.M., & Lip, G.Y. (2002). Psychological factors in heart failure: A review of the literature. *Archives of Internal Medicine, 162,* 51–61.

Melzak, R. (1990). The tragedy of needless pain. *Scientific American, 262,* 27–33.

Meyers, T.J., & Mark, M.M. (1995). Effects of psychosocial interventions on adult cancer patients. A meta-analysis of randomized experiments. *Health Psychology, 14,* 101–108.

Miller, J., Fletcher, K., et al. (1995). Three year follow-up and clinical implications of a mindfulness meditation-based stress reduction intervention in the treatment of anxiety disorders. *General Hospital Psychiatry, 17,* 192–200.

Mind-Body medicine news. (2005*). Advances, 21,* 33.

Morin, C.M., et al. (1999). A randomized controlled trial of stress reduction for hypertension in older African Americans. *Hypertension, 6,* 820–827.

Munro, S., and Mount, B. (1978) Music therapy in palliative care. *Cancer Medicine Association Journal, 119,* 1029–1034.

Nagarathna, R., & Nagendra, H.R. (1985). Yoga for bronchial asthma: A controlled study. *British Medical Journal Clinical Research ED, 291,* 1077–1079.

Nako, M., Nomaron, S., et al. (1997). Clinical effects of blood pressure biofeedback treatment on hypertension by auto shaping. *Psychosomatic Medicine, 59,* 331–338.

Nako, M., Nomura, S., Shimosawa, T., Fujita, T., & Kuboki, T. (1999). Blood pressure treatment, organ damage and sympathetic activity in mild hypertension. *Psychotherapy and Psychosomatics, 68,* 341–347.

Naomi, R. (1997). Kitchen table wisdom: A conversation that heals. *Alternative Therapies, 3.*

National Institutes of Health. (1992). *Alternative Medicine: Expanding Medical Horizons.* Washington, DC: U.S. Government Printing Office.

National Institutes of Health. (1993). New research frontiers in behavioral medicine. Washington, DC: U.S. Government Printing Office.

National Institutes of Health. Web site. Retrieved October 12, 1999.

NIH Fields of Practice. (1999, November). National Institutes of Health Web site. Retrieved from http://nccam.nib.gov/ncccom/what-is-cam/fields/mind.htm#meditation.

NIH/OAM Consensus Report, Panel 5 (1998).

Ornish, D. (2003) Toward a joyful life. *Advances, 19,* 23–25.

Ospina-Kammerer, V. & Dixon, D.R. (2001). Coping with burnout: Family physicians and family social workers—what do they have in common? *Journal of Family Social Work, 5,* 85–93.

Ospina-Kammerer, V. (1999). Poetry therapy within a therapist's practice model. *Human Sciences, 12* (3).

Ospina-Kammerer, V., & Figley, C. (2003). An evaluation of the Respiratory One Method (ROM) in reducing emotional exhaustion among family physician residents. *International Journal of Emergency Mental Health, 5* (1), 29–32.

Ostir, G. V. (2004). Onset of frailty in older adults and the protective role of positive affect. *Psychology and Aging, 19,* 402–408.

Palsson, O. (2006). The nature of IBS and the need for a psychological approach. *International Journal of Clinical and Experimental Hypnosis, 54,* 1–5.

Palsson, O.S. (2006). Standardized hypnosis treatment for irritable syndrome: The North Carolina protocol. *The International Journal of Clinical and Experimental Hypnosis, 54,* 51–64.

Palsson, O.S., Turner, M.J., Johnson, D.A., Burnett, C.K., & Whitehead, W.E. (2002). Hypnosis treatment for severe irritable bowel syndrome—Investigation of mechanism and effects on symptoms. *Digestive Diseases and Sciences, 47,* 2605–2614.

Patterson, D.R., Adcock, R.J., & Bombardier, C.H. (1997). Factors predicting hypnotic analgesia in clinical burn pain. *The International Journal of Clinical and Experimental Hypnosis, 55,* 377–395.

Pelletier, K. (2002). Mind as healer, mind as slayer: Mind Body medicine comes of age. *Advances, 18,* 4–13.

Pelletier, K.R. (2004). Mind-body medicine in ambulatory care. An evidence-based assessment. *Journal of Ambulatory Care Management, 27,* 25–42.

Pennebaker, J.W. (1997). *Opening Up: The Healing Power of Expressing Emotions.* New York: Guilford Press.

Pert, C. (1997). *Molecules of Emotion.* New York: Scribner.

Pert, C. (2002). The wisdom of the receptors: Neuropeptides, the emotions, and bodymind. *Advances, 18,* 30–34.

Pinus, T. (1994). Data confirm the social context of disease. *Advances, 10,* 2.

Plaut, S.M., & Friedman, S.M. (1981). Psychosocial factors in infectious disease. In R. Ader (Ed.), *Psychoneuroimmunology* (pp. 3–26). Orlando, FL: Academic Press.

Pliszka, S. (2003). *Neuroscience for the Mental Health Clinician.* New York: Guilford Press.

Polenghi, M.M., Molinari, E., Gala, C., Guzzi, R., Garutti, C., & Finzi, A.F. (1994). Experience with psoriasis in a psychosomatic dermatology clinic. *Acta Dermato-venereologica. Supplementum (Stockholm), 186,* 65–66.

Power, C., et al. (2001). Predictors of low back pain onset in a prospective British study. *American Journal of Public Health, 91,* 1671–1678.

Pressman, S., & Cohen, S. (May 24, 2005). Lonliness, social network size, immune response to influenza vaccine in college freshmen, *Health Psychology, 3,* 297–306.

Prinshorn. (1992). *Artistry of the Mentally Ill* in *Alternative Medicine: Expanding Medical Horizons.* (National Institutes of Health report). Washington, DC: U.S. Government Printing Office.

Quinn, J. (1989). Therapeutic touch as energy exchange: Replication and extension. *Nursing Science Quarterly, 12,* 78–87.

Rao, S., & Enck, P. (1997). Biofeedback therapy for defecation disorders. *Digestive Disorder, 15,* 78–92.

Raz, A. (2006). *Proceedings of the National Academy of Sciences, 102,* 9978–9983.

Read, N.W. (1999). Harnessing the patient's power. *Baillieres Best Practice and Research in Clinical Gastroenterology, 13,* 473–487.

Remington, R. (2002). Calming music and hand massage with agitated elderly. *Nursing Research, 51,* 317–323.

Report from Cleveland Clinic. (1997). *Mind/Body Newsletter,* 3.

Richardson, J.L., et al. (1990). Support group. *Journal of Clinical Oncology, 8,* 356–364.

Richardson, J.L., Shelton, D., et al. (1990). The effect of compliance with treatment in survival among patients with hematologic malignancy. *Journal of Clinical Oncology, 8,* 356–364.

Richardson, M.A., et al. (1997). Coping, life attitudes, and immune response to imagery and group support after breast cancer treatment. *Alternative Therapies in Health and Medicine, 3,* 62–70.

Richman, L., et al. (2005). Positive emotion and health: Going beyond the negative. *Health Psychology, 24,* 422–429.

Robinson, L.A., et al. (1990). Psychotherapy for the treatment of depression: Comparison review of outcome research. *Psychological Bulletin.*

Rodgers, L. (1995). Music for surgery. *Advances, 11,* 49–56.

Rohan, K.J., Lindsey, K.T., Roecklein, K.A., Lacy, T.J. (2004). Cognitive-behavioral therapy, light therapy, and their combination in treating seasonal affective disorder. *Journal of Affective Disorder, 80*(2-3), 273–283.

Rosengreen, A., et al. (2004). Coronary disease in relation to social support and social class in Swedish men: A 15-year follow-up in the study of men born in 1933. *European Heart Journal, 25,* 56–63.

Rossi, E., & Cheek, D. (1998). *Mind-Body Therapy: Methods of Ideodynamic Healing in Hypnosis.* New York: Norton.

Rossman, M. (1989). *Healing Yourself: A Step-by-Step Program for Better Health Through Imagery.* New York: Pocket Books.

Rossman, M. (1993). Imagery: Learning to use the mind's eye. In D. Goleman (Ed.), *Mind Body Medicine.* Yonkers, NY: Consumer Reports Books.

Ruguiles, R. (200). Depression as a predictor for coronary heart disease: A review and meta-analysis. *American Journal of Preventive Medicine, 23,* 51–61.

Rush, A. (1996). *The Modern Book of Yoga: Exercising Mind, Body, and Spirit.* New York: Bantam/Dell Publishing Group.

Ruske, S., Blecke, D., & Reinfraw, M. (2006). Cognitive therapy for depression. *American Family Physician, 73.*

Rutledge, T., & Hogan, B.E. (2002). A quantitative review of prospective evidence linking psychosocial factors with hypertension development. *Psychosomatic Medicine, 64,* 758–766.

Ruyylasmith, P., et al. (1995). Effects of hypnosis on the immune response: B-cells, T-cells, helper and suppressor cells. *American Journal of Clinical Hypnosis, 38,* 71–79.

Sabaawi, M. (2004). The mind and the brain: Neuroplasticity and the power of mental force. *Journal of Child and Family Studies,* 13, 125–127.

Sagan, C. (1985) *Cosmos.* New York: Ballantine Books.

Santorelli, S.F. (1999). *Heal Thyself, Lessons on Mindfulness in Medicine.* New York: Random House-Bell Tower.

Sarafine, E. (2000). Age comparison in acquiring biofeedback control and success in reducing headache pain. *Annals of Behavior Medicine, 2*, 10.

Schafer, W. (1996). *Stress Management for Wellness*. Fort Worth, TX: Harcourt Brace College Publishers.

Schafer, W. (1996). *Stress Management for Wellness*. Orlando, FL: Holt, Rinehart & Winston.

Schlitz, M., & Braud, W. (1997). Distant intentionality and healing: Assessing the evidence. *Alternative Therapies in Health and Medicine, 3*, 62–73.

Schneider, R.H., Staggters, F., et al. (1995). A randomized controlled trial of stress reduction for hypertension in older African Americans. *Hypertension, 26*, 820–827.

Schroeder-Sheker. (2006). *The Luminous Wound*. In press.

Schwartz, J.M., Stoessel, P.W., Baxter, Jr., L.R., Martin, K.M., & Phelps, M.E. (1996). Systematic changes in cerebral glucose metabolic rate after successful behavior modification treatment of obsessive-compulsive disorder. *Archives General Psychiatry, 53*, 109–113.

Schwartz, M., & Andrasick, F. (2006). *Biofeedback: A Practitioner's Guide*. New York: Guilford Press.

Schwartz & Schwartz. (1993). Biofeedback using the body signals. In Goleman & Gurin (Eds.), *Mind Body Medicine*. Yonkers, NY: Consumers Report Books.

Segal, Z. (2000). *Mindfulness Based Cognitive Therapy for Depression*. New York: Guilford Press.

Seligman, M.E., Steen, T., et al. (2005). Positive psychology progress: Empirical validation of interventions. *American Psychologist, 60*, 410–421.

Selye, H. (1936). *The Stress of Life*. New York: McGraw-Hill.

Selye, H. (1980). *Seyle's Guide to Stress Research*. New York: Van Nostrand Reinhold.

Shapiro, S.L., et al. (2001). Meditation and positive psychology. In C. R. Snyder and S. Lopex (Eds.). *Handbook of Positive Psychology*. Oxford, UK.

Shavit, Y., et al. (1985). Stress, opioid peptides, the immune system and cancer. *Journal of Immunology, 135*, 834–837.

Shenefelt, P.D. (2000). Hypnosis in dermatology. *Archives of Dermatology, 136*, 393–399.

Sheps, D.S., et al. (2002). Mental stress induced ischemia and all cause mortality in persons with coronary artery disease: Results in the psychophysiological investigations of myocardial ischemia study. *Circulation, 84*, 1780–1789.

Sherman, K.J., Cherkin, D.C., Erro, J., et al. (2005) Comparing yoga, exercise, and a self-care book for chronic bow back pain: a randomized, controlled trial. *Annals of Internal Medicine, 143*, 849–856.

Sicher, F., et al. (1998). A randomized double-blind study of the effects of distant healing in a population of advanced AIDS. *Western Journal of Medicine, 169*, 356–363.

Siegal, B. (2003). Healing our lives. *Advances, 19*, 13–14.

Sierpina, V. (2001). *Integrative Health Care: Complementary and Alternative Therapies for the Whole Person*. Philadelphia: Davis.

Slattery, D. P. (1999). Poetry, prayer and meditation. *Journal of Poetry Therapy, 13*, 39–45.

Smith, M., & Perles, M. (2006). Who is a candidate for cognitive-behavioral therapy for insomnia? *Health Psychology, 25*, 15–19.

Smith, R.S. (1991). The immune system is a key factor in the etiology of psychosocial disease. *Medical Hypnosis, 34*, 49–57.

Smith, R.W., et al. (2002). Psychosocial influences on the development and course of coronary heart disease: Current status and implications for practice and research. *Journal of Consulting and Clinical Psychology, 70*, 548–568.

Smyth, J.M. (1998). Written emotional expression: Effect size, outcome types, and moderating variables. *Journal of Counseling and Clinical Psychology, 66,* 174–184.

Smyth, J.M., et al. (1999). Effect of writing about stressful experiences on symptom reduction in patients with asthma and rheumatoid arthritis: A randomized trial. *Journal of the American Medical Association, 14* (281), 1304–1309.

Sobel, R.K. (2006). Does laughter make good medicine? *New England Journal of Medicine, 16,* 1114–1115.

Solomon, F. G. (1997). Clinical and social implications of stress-induced neuro-endocrine-immune interactions. In J. C. Buckingham, G. E. Gillies, & A. M. Cowell (Eds.), *Stress, Stress Hormones and the Immune System* (pp. 385–401). New York: Wiley.

Speca, M., et al. (2000). A randomized wait list controlled clinical trial: the effect of a mind fullness meditation-based reduction program on mood symptoms of stress in cancer outpatients, *Psychosomatic Medicine, 62* (5), 613–622.

Spiegel, D. (1998). Support group. *Public Health Reports, 110,* 298.

Spiegel, D. (1999). Healing words: Emotional expression and disease outcome. *Journal of the American Medical Association, 281,* 1328–1329.

Spiegal, D., et al. (1989). Effect of psychosocial treatment of survival of patients with metastatic breast cancer. *Lancet, 2,* 888–891.

Spielberger, C.D., Gorsuch, R.L., et al. (1998). *Manual for the State-Trait Anxiety Inventory*. Palo Alto, CA: Consulting Psychologists Press.

Spira, M., & Carlson, L. (2000). *Psychosomatic Medicine, 62* (5), 318–320.

Steegmans, Paul H.A., et al. (2000). Higher prevalence of depressive symptoms in middle-aged men with low serum cholesterol levels. *Psychomatic Medicine, 62*, 205–211.

Sternberg, P. (2001). Drama therapy. In N. Allison (Ed.), *The Complete Body, Mind, Spirit* (pp. 318–320). New York: McGraw-Hill.

Stolbach, L (2003). Does fighting spirit improve medical outcomes of cancer patients? *Advances, 19*, 17–18.

Sung Dell, R.H., et al. (2000). *American Journal of Hypertension, 13,* 185A–186A.

Surwit, R. (2004). *The Mind-Body Diabetes Revolution*. New York: Free Press.

Syrjala, K.L., et al. (1995) Relaxation and imagery and cognitive-behavioral training reduce pain during cancer treatment: A controlled clinical trial. *Pain, 63,* 189–198.

Targ, E., & Taylor, S.E. (2001). Prayer and distant healing positive and negative beliefs and the course of AIDS. *Advances in Mind-Body Medicine, 17,* 2.

Teastate, J.D. (2002). Relapse-recurrence in major depression by mindfulness based cognitive therapy. *Journal of Consulting and Clinical Psychology, 68*, 615–623.

Thase, M.E., & Howland, R.H. (1994). Refractory depression: Relevance of psychosocial factors and therapies. *Psychiatry Annals, 24*, 232–240.

Theorell, T. (2005). *Journal of Epidemiology and Community Health, 59*, 23–30.

Tusek, D., Church, J., et al. (1997): Guided imagery. A significant advance in the care of patients undergoing elective colorectal surgery. *Diseases of the Colon and Rectum, 40*, 172–178.

Ulrich, P.M., & Lutgendorf, S.K. (2002). Journaling about stressful events: Effects of cognitive processing and emotional expression. *The Society of Behavioral Medicine, 24.*

Van Kampen, M., et al. (2000). Effect of pelvic-floor re-education on duration and degree of incontinence after radical prostatectomy: A randomized controlled trial. *Lancet, 355*, 98–102.

Van Melle, J.P., de Jonge, P., et al. (2004). Prognostic association for depression following myocardial infarction with mortality and cardiovascular events: A meta-analysis. *Psychosomatic Medicine, 66*, 814–882.

Van Talden, M. W., et al. (2000). Analysis of research. *Spine, 26*, 270–281.

Vathera, J., & Kivimaki, N. (2004). *British Medical Journal.*

Vedanthan, P., et al. (1998). Clinical study of yoga techniques in university students with asthma. A controlled study. *Allergy Asthma Procedure, 19*, 3–9.

Walker, L.G., et al. Psychological, clinical and pathological effects of relaxation training and guided imagery during primary chemotherapy. *British Journal of Cancer, 80*, 262–268.

Wang, S.M. (2002). Music and preoperative anxiety. A randomized controlled study. *Journal of Anesthesia and Analgesia, 94*, 1489–1494.

Wassertheil-Smoller, S. (2004). Depression and cardiovascular sequelae in postmenopausal women. *Archives of Internal Medicine, 164*, 289–298.

Watson, D., & Hubbard, B. (1996). Adaptational style and dispositional structure: Coping in the context of the five-factor model. *Journal of Personality, 64* (4), 737.

Weil, A. (1997). *Eight Weeks to Optimum Health.* New York: Random House.

Whitehead, W. (2006). Hypnosis for irritable bowel syndrome: The empirical evidence of therapeutic effects. *The International Journal of Clinical and Experimental Hypnosis, 54* (1), 7–20.

Williams, K., Petroni, J., Smith, D., et al. (2005). Effect of Iyengar yoga therapy for chronic low back pain. *Pain, 115*, 107–117.

Wilson, S.R., & Scamages, P. (1993). A controlled trial of two forms of self-management education for adults with asthma. *American Journal of Medicine. 94*, 564–576.

Wilson, R.S. (2003). Proneness to psychological distress is associated with risk of Alzheimer's disease. *Neurology, 61*, 1479–1485.

Winterowed, C., Beck, A., et al. (2003). *Cognitive Therapy With Chronic Pain Patients.* New York: Springer.

Wirth, D. (1990). The effect of non-contact therapeutic touch on the healing rate of full-thickness surgical wounds. *Subtle Energies, 1*, 1–20.

Yan, L.L., et al. (2003). Psychosocial factors and risk of hypertension: The coronary artery and risk development study in young adults (Cardia) study. *Journal of the American Medical Association, 22*, 290, 2136–2148.

Yung, P.M., et al. (2002). A controlled trial of music and pre-operative anxiety in Chinese men undergoing transurethral resection of the prostate. *Journal of Advanced Nursing, 39*, 352–359.

Zutra, A., et al. (1989). Life stress and lymphocyte alterations among patients with rheumatoid arthritis. *Health Psychology, 8*, 1–14.

Index

Made in the USA
Monee, IL
13 September 2026

62976819R00107